CHANGE YOUR
DIET
CHANGE YOUR
HEALTH

HOW FOOD CAN MAINTAIN OUR HEALTH
OR CAUSE DISEASE

Jorge Bordenave MD FACP

Integrative Cardiologist

authorHOUSE®

AuthorHouse™
1663 Liberty Drive
Bloomington, IN 47403
www.authorhouse.com
Phone: 1-800-839-8640

Published by AuthorHouse   03/24/2012

ISBN: 978-1-4567-9510-8 (sc)
ISBN: 978-1-4567-9509-2 (hc)
ISBN: 978-1-4567-9507-8 (e)

Library of Congress Control Number: 2011915770

Dedication

This book is dedicated to all those who would like to learn how to take better control of their health, without so many medicines or relying on our Nations broken healthcare system.

To my father, Carlos, a family physician who set a high bar for me to follow, and my mother, Odilia, a PhD in education, who was always ahead of her time.

For my esposa, for helping me become a better, healthier and more compassionate physician. She is a constant reminder of natures' beauty.

"The doctor of the future will prescribe no medicine, but will want to educate their patients in the care of the body, proper diet, and disease prevention."

~ Thomas A. Edison

Contents

PART 2

Preface

This book is a translation from the original Spanish text, "La dieta anti-inflammatoria" (The Anti-Inflammatory Diet), Balboa Press.

It was written because your health and wellbeing is important to me, as well as those who care about you.

When I first started my solo cardiology practice, I was in my early thirties and most, if not all of the patients I was treating were older than me. The typical office consultations were for problems relating to high blood pressure, high cholesterol, coronary artery disease, ischemic heart diseases, chest pain and various other cardiovascular diseases, that are normally associated with an older demographic. With time, however, I began seeing younger patients suffering from various cardiovascular conditions, as well as complications associated with chronic disease. An increase in chronic disease affecting young patients that in large part resulted because of poor nutritional choices and sedentary lifestyles.

While I was seeing a steady increase in younger aged patients with multiple and more complex health issues, I was also growing older and I started to realize just how lucky I had been with my health. I also realized I had been taking my health for granted.

The steady stream of younger aged patients continued. I was treating an ever-growing number of young adults in their twenties, thirties and forties who were coming in for evaluation while already being on combination drug therapy (consisting of blood pressure medications, cholesterol medications, sleeping pills, anxiety medications, anti-depressants, and stomach acid suppressing medications). The one thing that many of these young patients shared in common was the fact that they were overweight.

This was due to their energy dense diets, which consisted of high calorie fast foods and snacks, little or no exercise or physical activity, and a lack of interest in the care of their own health. These were the same characteristics and qualities that have been typical of our American way of life over the last decades. This was very concerning to me.

During this time, I was also noticing that a great majority of the hospitalized patients I was consulting were struggling with end stage complications of common chronic illnesses that could have been easily prevented, if only they had exercised a little self-care.

The majority of these hospitalized patients were now suffering from the results of years of poor lifestyle choices that many of us (including myself), take for granted, and which mainly come in the form of bad dietary choices, poor nutrition, and sedentary lives.

Patients who had become debilitated, weak and frail—many with multiple systemic problems and poor quality of life, who were hooked up to machines that act only in prolonging death instead of preserving health or restoring quality of life.

This got me thinking that despite our current understanding of health and the millions of dollars spent on campaigns to teach and educate people on the importance of nutrition and exercise, many of us still do not take care of ourselves. We are either in denial, misinformed or of the belief that we need not have to work to preserve our health.

I, too, had become lazy and admit to having found myself in this last category. I would go to the gym to work out, but only so that I could eat as much food as I wanted, which mostly consisted of highly processed, poor quality, and high caloric foods. This was similar to the habits of the majority of the patients I treated, who did not see any urgency in changing their lifestyle choices until they were sitting in my examining room, consumed by anxiety. For whatever reason, we seem to put off and postpone taking care of ourselves until it is too late.

We live our lives believing we are well, while we slowly transition from wellness to illness. I think it is fair to say that many of us are so busy with all that life throws at us that we don't realize the extent to which many of us will become ill.

The severity of that illness often times depends on our lifestyle choices.

When we do become ill, we assume and believe that there will be medications that will cure us and doctors that will take care of us. Why shouldn't we believe this? We live in a world where even the most serious illnesses are cured in less than an hour every week on episodes of "House", "Grey's Anatomy" and other popular TV shows. This is the CSI effect applied to healthcare: Everything has a scientifically explainable cause and quick resolution.

While many people spend thousands of dollars on procedures and therapies that fight the aging process on the outside, they neglect the most important part of the body and soul, which is located on the inside. Our internal organs, blood vessels, and most importantly, our psyche and our mental health are usually overlooked.

Food and nutrition play a vital role in maintaining health, wellness and balance, and are important factors that contribute to how you look on the outside and feel on the inside.

The fact that many care more about and focus on how they look on the outside rather than how they feel on the inside has to do with the fact that many of us in the general public, as well as the medical field, know very little when it comes to nutrition and diet. It is also because we have become a society that is accustomed to instant gratification: We want and expect quick fixes for just about everything, including the improvement of our looks.

The increasing number of younger aged patients with serious medical illnesses was my wake up call. It got me thinking about how lucky I am for being as healthy as I am. The hospitalized patients gave me an insight into my possible future if I chose to continue abusing my body with poor food choices and half-hearted exercise (which I was doing for the all the wrong reasons).

I sought out and learned about nutrition during my third Fellowship at the University of Arizona Center for Integrative Medicine. For the first time in my many years of formal medical training, continuing medical education and career, I was taught and learned about the importance of food and nutrition in maintaining and restoring health.

Because I had learned so much, and love teaching and empowering my patients, I started sharing my newfound knowledge with them. It was my patients who suggested that I write a book and that is exactly what I did.

My continuing study and research for this book, has definitely made me see food and nutrition as an important and integral component of health and wellness. It is a topic importance and relevance and that must be taught in medical schools.

Hopefully this book will serve as your wake up call or at the very least, offer insight on the importance of food and nutrition in your life and the lives of those you love.

The information contained in this book is current and truly fascinating. You will find information that will be new to most people, including doctors, because it is material that most physicians, including myself, were never trained in or learned during our medical school or residency training. This is especially true in regards to the relation that exists between our nutrition, diet, and the development of various common chronic diseases.

What it all boils down to is our lifestyle choices.

We can continue to ignore taking care of ourselves and wait for chronic multi-organ damage, to occur followed by a lifetime of limitations and medications, or we can be a little bit more aware of what we put in our bodies and learn to make better choices. It is *that* simple.

I wish that everyone had an opportunity to walk with me down hospital corridors, into patient rooms, and through the intensive care units so they could see their potential future, should they choose to continue on their current path.

This is what I think about when I see patients hooked up to machines. And frankly, it is terrifying.

If you are healthy, regardless of your age, thank God for it and take care of it. Don't push your luck or wait to become another statistic, because unfortunately, many of us will.

Avoid being a hospitalized patient at all costs, at the mercy of our broken health care system. A system that to many, feels robotic, sterile and relies too heavily on drugs, pills and tests. Many of us are living longer and it is a natural process for the functions of our bodies to deteriorate and decline with age and time. We can, however, improve our bodies' natural functions and help slow down this natural decline with the foods we eat. Genes are important for longevity, but nutrition is a central component within our control for maintaining health.

Obesity related diseases, as well as many chronic diseases develop as a result of poor nutritional choices and causes an acceleration of the normal functional decline. We can't control the genes we inherit, but why not control factors we can?

All of us need to be pro-active and take care of our own health, so that we can stay healthy and enjoy a good quality of life well into our 90's instead of being on multiple medications by the age of 20.

The good news is that you can slow down and even reverse many of our common chronic illnesses by taking better care of your body, learning to eat healthier, staying active, and changing our lifestyle.

Health is the great equalizer.

Acknowledgements

First and foremost, I would like to thank and acknowledge all of my colleagues of the 2011 Summer Class of the University of Arizona Center for Integrative Medicine.

Never before had I had the honor of meeting, and being associated with such a diverse group of caring and compassionate physicians from all over the world.

These were individuals of different ages, cultures, traditions and disciplines who where brought together at a particular moment in time to graduate with the understanding that healing is an inherent quality of all living organisms.

In our differences, we recognize just how alike we all are.

A special thanks to Dr. Andrew Weil, Dr. Tieraona Low Dog, Dr. Randy Horwitz, Dr. Victoria Maizes, Moira, Tanya and everyone else who guided our journey and lead us to a continued path of exploration.

Kindred spirits.

We are all, always family.

Valeria Manavello, for editing the manuscript.

Finally, a very special thanks to my esposa and nutritionist Billie Smith, who completed her nutrition degree at Florida International University in Miami, and who has taught me most of what I know about nutrition. She was instrumental in the production of this book and I am lucky to have her free help, before she becomes a well known and highly sought after, diet and nutrition personality. Thank you for being u.

Te amo.

PART ONE

Disease, Inflammation, and Our Nutrition

The concept of chronic, persistent inflammation as a cause of chronic diseases has been around for over 200 years. However, it has only been within the last decade or so however, that we have been able to better understand the multiple, complex, biochemical and physiologic interactions that occur in the pathophysiology of systemic inflammation and how they relate to disease development.

Evidence has shown, and continues to support, inflammation as the root cause of many of today's common illnesses and medical conditions.

There is also evidence that suggests that certain types of environmental toxins, acquired either while developing in utero, after birth, or perhaps more importantly, as a result of the foods that we have been consuming as part of a "Western" type diet, contribute directly to the development of inflammation and systemic pro-inflammatory states.

Continuous consumption of foods that are highly refined, processed, and that contain large quantities of saturated and trans fat, or that have been exposed to chemicals or trans-fats during their manufacturing process, that can lead to persistent, long-lasting, low grade inflammation.

Awareness of these facts has the potential of allowing us to make better food and lifestyle choices, which can reverse the discouraging health trends our country has been facing for several decades.

What we eat really makes a difference in our health, making the old adage, "you are what you eat" more relevant than ever.

This is especially true at the start of the 21st century. Despite our successes and impressive advances in medicine, our country leads the world in epidemics of obesity and lifestyle related illnesses (such as diabetes, heart disease, strokes, cancers, digestive disorders, and even mood and cognitive mental disorders). Chronic medical conditions that are occurring at younger ages and continue for a lifetime are important contributors for our escalating, out of control healthcare costs.

According to the Centers for Disease Control and Prevention (CDC), 32% of white women and 53% of black women are obese. In 2007, almost 11% of adults over 20 years had might find this surprising, or maybe even hadn't considered food as a drug.

One definition of "drug" is: Any substance that, when absorbed into the body of a living organism, alters normal bodily function.

Doesn't food do this? Not only that, most of us consume food in a ritualistic manner at least three times a day. Over our lifetime, food, its quality, consistency and quantity, as well as everything that went into producing it, is vitally important to our health and wellbeing.

Food has been utilized as a drug and as medicine in traditional Chinese medicine (TCM), Ayurvedic medicine of India, the medicine of the ancient Roman Empire, and of Egyptian and South American cultures—all of which date back thousands of years before Christ.

While growing up, how many of us didn't feel relief and got better quicker from a cold, after a bowl or cup of mom's homemade chicken soup?

A few years ago an article was even published confirming the fact that hot soup did in fact help alleviate cold symptoms quicker.

"Feed a cold, starve a fever" is a common saying in the lexicon of Americana. Or is it the other way around? Regardless, diabetes, while 23% of all individuals over the age of 60 had diabetes (http://www.cdc.gov/diabetes/pubs/pdf/ndfs_2007.pdf).

Healthcare costs in 2008, the latest year which monetary figures are available, totaled $2.3 trillion dollars ($2.300,000,000,000.00), or 20% of this nation's Gross Domestic Product (GDP). By comparison, in 1980 our nations healthcare expenditure was $247 billion, or 8.8% of our GDP (www.ncbi.nlm.nih.gov/pubmed/10309470).

Five common medical conditions are responsible for more than half of this country's total health care expenditures, as well as for two-thirds of the total amount of money paid out t Medicare (Druss et al 2001).

These are five medical conditions that can be controlled and in many instances reversed, simply by changing our diets and increasing our activity level.

These five include: cardiovascular disorders, obesity, diabete pulmonary diseases and cancer.

While genetic and hereditary factors are causes of some diseases and are out of our control, there are many other factors that we can control in order to lessen our chances of developing diseases and becoming ill.

Food is, and has always been, the single most important medication we utilize during our journey throughout life. Ma whether we remember it or acknowledge it, food has played an important role in health and disease.

Most of us today, are aware of some negative food-disease associations, such as the consumption of saturated fats with the development of cardiovascular disease or of weight gain, and obesity, and the development of diabetes with increased carbohydrate consumption. The elimination of foods that contain wheat protein is the mainstay treatment of the under-diagnosed condition called "Celiac Disease" or "gluten insensitivity". Likewise, the withholding of food items (which will be mentioned in later in later chapters) serve as a key treatment component of many other illnesses that share an established food-disease association.

More importantly, many of us forget, take for granted, or are even unaware of the positive associations of food with our health. Epidemiological studies have shown that diets that are high in fruits and vegetables and low in meats containing saturated fats have consistently resulted in lower cancer risks.

It has been estimated that approximately 35% of all cancers in the United States have a potential diet related association, surpassing smoking as a risk factor (Doll R, Peto R. The causes of cancer: quantitative estimates of avoidable risks of cancer in the United States today. Journal of the National Cancer Institute 66(6):1191-308 Jun, 1981).

This fact, for me, is just amazing and eye opening.

Many of us may not be aware that Alzheimer's disease and dementia progression can be slowed by the diet we consume, or that a lipoprotein (a type of fat) called apoE 4, which is measured in the blood, has been associated with a higher risk for the development of Alzheimer's disease. These are just a few of the many associations that exists between the foods we have been eating and are still eating today, with the development of many of the most common diseases we suffer from.

Lack of physical activity, movement and exercise compounds and adds to the disease/illness scenario.

I wrote this book to make people aware of this.

There is such an overload of recommendations, diets, fads, weight loss gimmicks, unsubstantiated health claims and misinformation that even I still get confused with all the health claims being made!

The bottom line is your food selection is not only responsible for your weight, but more importantly, it is responsible for your health.

So choose wisely.

For example, whenever we cut ourselves or sustain any other type of injury, within a few milliseconds an inflammatory chain of events, better known as an inflammatory cascade, becomes activated. Damage to the membranes of cells release various chemicals that will trigger an escalating inflammatory response, depending on the need. Some of these chemicals are products of arachidonic acid metabolism, and include substances like prostaglandins and leukotrienes, as well as bradikinins and histamins. All of these have important functions in the acute inflammatory response. Mainly, they increase and create more inflammation.

These chemical mediators cause an increased blood flow to the site of injury and are typically the cause of the initial localized pain associated with an acute inflammatory process. The increase flow of blood and fluid into the injured area causes swelling, and the increased dilation of the blood vessels causes redness.

Eventually, the immune system may become activated by a process called chemotaxis, in which white blood cells arrive at the site of injury. A key inflammatory activator is a molecule called Nf-kappa B. This molecule acts as a signal to turn up the body's inflammatory response, which in turn causes an increased release of other pro-inflammatory chemicals such as intrleukin-6 (IL-6), interleukin 1L-beta, tumor necrosis factor alpha, and cyclo-oxygenase-2 (COX-2). All of these chemicals

Understanding Inflammation.

It is becoming more evident that inflammation plays a vital role in the development of many wide-ranging chronic illnesses.

Inflammation is a normal bodily process that serves to keep us healthy. It is our body's principal defense response mechanism to infection, injury or any noxious stimuli. We need an intact and adequately functioning inflammatory system to maintain wellness and to stay healthy throughout life.

Inflammatory processes are a common defense response of the body, occurring hundreds of times throughout the day in order to protect us against invading organisms and processes that can potentially cause us harm. When the threat is neutralized, the inflammatory process turns itself off and remains on alert, ready for any future injury or noxious stimuli.

Acute inflammation is an immediate, overwhelming and short-acting response to a trauma, irritation, endo-toxin (chemicals), bacteria, viruses, microorganisms and other potentially damaging stimulus.

are important components of a normal inflammatory response. However, they also play a role in chronic diseases.

Neutrophils are the white blood cells responsible in finding and eliminating any bacteria. They do so by engulfing or swallowing these microorganisms and destroying them with potent enzymes within its cell structure. Neutrophils, which have a very short life of several hours, are assisted in the removal of cellular debris by macrophages, another type of white blood cell.

Depending on the type of injury, the hematologic system may also be activated, with platelets quickly clumping together, forming localized blood clots that stop and prevent any potential bleeding.

In addition to these blood cell components, the injured area is also flooded with other anticoagulant factors and chemicals that work together to protect the body from the injury.

In a healthy person, this response to injury or infection is quick and efficient, with resolution occurring before the immune system is chronically activated. This is how normal inflammation should occur: As a temporary, limited process that turns itself on and shuts itself off.

An immediate, short-lasting response that ends quickly after the elimination of the triggering threat is typical of an acute inflammation process. Occasionally, we are aware of it because it occurs as a result of a direct injury or trauma in a superficial or exposed area that we can see and feel directly.

Anyone who has ever cut themselves or suffered a skin abrasion (scrape) from a fall, knows that after the initial pain, swelling and redness, resulting from this acute inflammatory process is contained and resolved, the skin eventually returns to its normal color and temperature.

Another example of an acute inflammatory response occurs with a flare up of gout. Gout is a condition of altered uric acid metabolism where there is too much uric acid in the body. As these uric acid levels increase, they may precipitate and form crystals that are frequently deposited in the fluids and lining around the joints. These crystals cause the surrounding area to become irritated, which causes an inflammatory process to begin. This process is manifested by redness, swelling, and pain or tenderness to the affected area, frequently localized in one joint.

A more common example of an acute inflammatory process is that of a common head cold. A red and runny nose, watering eyes, and perhaps pain around the sinuses in the face are all products of the acute localized inflammatory response that causes blood vessels to dilated, swell up and increase fluid flow to the area.

More importantly, many of us are unaware that the illness, medical condition or disease process that we, or someone we care about, suffer from are a form of chronic inflammation.

Other examples of chronic inflammation include: atherosclerosis or hardening of the arteries, peptic ulcer disease, psoriasis, rheumatoid arthritis, pancreatitis, Alzheimer's disease, inflammatory bowel disease, allergies, obesity, cancer, diabetes, asthma as well as many others. By the diversity of these illnesses, one can see that chronic inflammation is an increasingly common factor in many diverse diseases.

A hundred years ago, high doses of aspirin and aspirin-containing medications were used to lower glucose levels in diabetics. To many, this suggested a probable association between inflammation and diabetes. It was only recently shown, however, that the reason aspirin lowered glucose levels is by simulating an immunologic component of insulin resistance that can occur in non-insulin dependant diabetes (Vol 116, Issue 7, July 3, 2006 J Clin Invest. 116(7):1793-1801).

A study from the Mayo Clinic (reported at the American Academy of Allergy, Asthma and Immunology in San Francisco, March 2011), reviewed medical records from the late 1960's and found higher rates of diabetes and heart disease amongst asthmatics, as well as a similar positive association between rheumatoid arthritis and inflammatory bowel disease. Experts

In contrast to an acute inflammatory response, a chronic low-level inflammation is a persistent inflammation due to chronic irritation by exposure to a noxious stimuli or an autoimmune reaction.

Instead of neutrophils and macrophage responding to the site of injury, other types of white blood cells, in the form of monocytes, lymphocytes and fibroblasts will typically predominate. As this inflammation becomes chronic and continues indefinitely, other components of the body's defens system become activated. The compliment system is activated to aid antibodies and phagocytic cells in removal of noxious stimuli. Phagocytic cells are a type of cell, capable of engulfing or swallowing up and destroying invading cells. They also generate and produce many enzymes and chemicals, includir reactive oxygen species. These reactive oxygen species are pro-inflammatory and contribute to the cycle of chronic inflammation.

The coagulation system is activated to limit bleeding, by forming a network of fine protein strands that localize in the injured area. This is how thrombus, (a blood clot, as well as the main cause of sudden death and frequent cause of acute coronary syndromes) forms.

The body's complex protein system, or Kinin system, is activated and functions as an inflammatory mediator, causir even more vasodilatation. Finally, the fibrinolysis system were surprised at these findings because of the different immune profiles associated with these diverse groups of illnesses. But this is yet another example of an inflammatory relation, shared by and between many seemingly different medical conditions.

We know that persistent, low-grade inflammation exists because we can measure and quantify levels of bio-inflammatory markers in individuals, even when they lack typical symptoms of inflammation.

Biochemical marker elevations include: interleukin-6 (IL-6), C-reactive protein (hs-CRP), fibrinogen, tumor necrosis factor alpha, cytokines, erythrocyte sedimentation levels, IL-1, circulating levels of adiponectins, as well as other components and by-products of inflammation. Many of these biomarkers can also be encountered in acute inflammation. However, they return to normal once the acute inflammatory process is resolved.

Just as chronic inflammation can cause stimulation of our immune system, many immune system disorders can result in abnormal levels of inflammation, which stimulate the inflammatory cascade.

Inflammation is a normal and common bodily process that we have all had at one time or another. This is why some of the consistently top selling, over the counter medications in the country are anti-inflammatory medications. These include all aspirin products, as well as non-steroidal anti-inflammatory medications (NSAID's). NSAIDS include: celecoxib(Celebrex®), diclofenac sodium(Voltaren®), difiunisal(Dolobid®), ibuprofen(Advil®, Motrin®), indomethacin, meloxicam(Mobic®), naproxen sodium(Aleve®), rofecoxib(Vioxx®) and many more.

Inflammation that tends to be long lasting, chronic, that results from, or that is associated with an immunologic process often requires stronger anti-inflammatory medications that may include steroids, and even immunosuppressant drugs.

These work by blocking several of the chemical mediators involved in the immune process. When inflammation affects a joint severely enough to result in joint destruction, joint replacement surgery may be the only option available.

It is now widely accepted that chronic inflammation is the main cause in the process of atherosclerosis, rather than cholesterol build up. Atherosclerosis results in coronary artery disease, as well as a host of other common cardio-vascular disorders.

Inflammation as the cause of atherosclerosis is far from being a new concept, as it was first described by Dr. Rudolf Virchow more than 150 years ago in his book *Cellular Pathology as Based upon Physiological and Pathological History.*

Because this inflammatory process contributes to atherosclerosis, we physicians usually recommend an aspirin a day for most individuals at risk for heart disease. Aspirin acts to prevent the platelets (part of the coagulation system) from sticking together and forming clots in inflamed tissues. It is the same reason why aspirin and other anti-platelet medications are also routinely prescribed to patients who have had a stent placed, which help maintain the coronary artery open.

A frequently checked inflammatory marker in cardiology is C-reactive protein or high sensitivity CRP (hs-CRP). This substance circulates in the blood, and is present in several inflammatory conditions, including coronary artery disease. It is used to measure the different levels or intensities of inflammation associated with coronary artery disease.

C-reactive protein (CRP) is produced in the liver as a response to any inflammatory process, so it is not specific to heart disease. People with arthritis, collagen diseases, and other conditions associated with high levels of inflammation can also have elevated CRP levels.

Studies done on people with cardiac risk factors however, have shown an increased risk of cardiovascular and neurological disorders, including stroke, with elevated levels of CRP.

One of the first studies that established a link between inflammation and heart disease was published in 1997. The study found that baseline CRP measurements were able to predict the future risk of heart attack and stroke in seemingly healthy men between the ages of 40 and 84. This study also described a reduction in the rate of first heart attack with regular aspirin use—a finding that was directly related to the measured levels of CRP (N Engl J Med 1997; 336:973-979 April 3 1997).

The medical literature is full of studies and investigations that recommend checking CRP levels on all patients with risk factors for coronary heart disease, especially those without symptoms. This enables physicians to assess their levels of inflammation and better enable them to take a more aggressive control over their treatment.

An interesting concept proposed by some investigators is that cholesterol may in fact not be the cause of heart and cardio-vascular disease. Instead, the finding of varying levels of cholesterol elevation may be a response to the different intensities of inflammation that all these processes share in common.

They postulate that cholesterol may actually be responding to areas of the endothelium (a cell layer lining the walls of the arteries), creating a defensive, protective barrier in response to the elevated levels of inflammation, in an attempt to limit and control the inflammatory process.

rphic

ng the
sing
d not a
hanism
the

ve
auses.
ctors,
king

s

ed

ave elevated cholesterol
ree or levels of inflammation.
ted levels of cholesterol as a
cardiovascular disease, it may
erol level is an important and
as a marker for the true cause of
on.

ar level, especially in the endothelial
all, is an important reason why we
rol reducing statin drugs. The statin
t widely recognized and prescribed
ents sold in the United States. They are
as simvastatin (Zocor ®), atorvastatin,
n (Crestor ®), pravastatin (Pravachol®)

patients, I always recommend diet
s a first step in treating elevated lipids.
have an important role in the medical
tients.

levels of the different lipids (fats) that make
he primary indication of statin drugs, these
work by reducing inflammation at the level of
l wall.

This inflammation reducing effect is called the pleom[...] effect.

It is thought that it is this pleomorphic effect, in reduci[...] level of inflammation of the endothelial lining, and cau[...] subsequent stabilization of the cellular membranes (ar[...] direct reduction of cholesterol levels per se), is the me[...] responsible for producing the greatest positive effect o[...] statin class of drugs.

Statins are currently recommended and prescribed for [...] individuals with a history of heart disease, heart attacks[...] strokes, or who have a family history of heart disease (e[...] their cholesterol levels are in the normal range). Their e[...] are so important, that they are included as one of the sta[...] discharge medications given to individuals leaving the h[...] after a cardiac event (such as a heart attack or coronary [...] syndrome).

Alzheimer's disease and other forms of decreased cogniti[...] neurologic functioning have many possible contributing [...] These include genetic factors, as well as environmental fa[...] such as diabetes, exercise and physical activity levels, smo[...] history, diet, nutrition and others that are modifiable.

However, Alzheimer's disease is also thought to start out a[...] an inflammatory process. A study published in 2008 in the[...] journal Neurology (Neurology May 6, 2008 70:1672-1677), revea[...]

a 24% reduction in the risk of Alzheimer's disease in patients who had been taking the non-steroidal, anti-inflammatory pain medication ibuprofen for a period greater than 5 years. The typical amyloid plaques, characteristic of this disease, start forming years before symptoms develop. They may develop as a response to underlying levels of inflammation, much like cholesterol is believed to develop in the atherosclerotic process.

Another common finding in Alzheimer's disease is the so-called neurofibrillary tangles, which consists of protein-like deposits that develop inside neurons. Although the exact trigger mechanism for the development of Alzheimer's is unknown, free radical formation and inflammation are known to play a pivotal role in its pathology (Farlow, Martin R. CONTINUUM: Lifelong Learning in Neurology Neurol 2007;13(2):39-68).

It is thought that this particular NSAID reduces inflammation and slows down and prevents the development of this disease in some patients.

Several studies have also shown a modest inverse association between chronic use of non-steroidal, anti-inflammatory drugs and the development of prostate cancer (Platz EA, et, Nonsteroidal anti-inflammatory drugs and risk of prostate cancer in the Baltimore Longitudinal Study of Aging. American Association for Cancer Research, cosponsored by the al. American Society of Preventive Oncology 14(2):390-6 Feb, 2005).

The development of some colon rectal cancers have also been associated with chronic inflammation of the digestive tract, as research has shown that regular use of non-steroidal, anti-inflammatory drugs lowers risk for colorectal adenomas (Hermann S, Rohrmann S, Linseisen J. Lifestyle factors, obesity and the risk of colorectal adenomas in EPIC-Heidelberg. Cancer causes & control : CCC 20(8):1397-408 Oct, 2009).

These examples are meant to highlight underlying inflammatory process as a common finding in what on the surface appears to be unrelated diseases.

They are not an endorsement of the prolonged use of a medication. No one should take a potentially toxic drug like a NSAID for prolonged periods.

Aging

When it comes to aging, is inflammation also a cause of aging, or is inflammation a response of the aging process?

There are many claims and many theories, but as of yet, there is no conclusive, definitive proof of an accepted, single mechanism for the aging process.

As of 2011, most papers and studies point to aging as being the end result of multiple factors. Inflammation is one of these factors, but not the sole cause.

According to work done at the University of Southern California by neurobiologist Caleb Finch, longevity was directly related to exposure to childhood diseases. Children born during times of high infectious burden resulted in higher inflammatory burden in adulthood, leading to shorter lives. Inflammation at a young age results in inflammation later in life, and impacts a person's lifespan (http://cmbi bjmu.edu.cn/news/0512/117.htm).

Other studies have related aging to inflammation based on the fact that many medical conditions have traditionally been associated with advancing age. Examples of these conditions include: Alzheimer's disease, osteoporosis, osteoarthritis, diabetes, muscle wasting diseases and obesity. Again, seemingly different medical conditions that share in common, chronic inflammation as an underlying cause.

Further studies postulate that aging is the final stage after a long-term accumulation of damage from repeated episodes of acute inflammation, or a result of a gradual shift from a cellular immunity pathway to one favoring a humoral immunity, as evidenced by reduced T-cell function (immune related) (National Institute on Aging, Workshop on Inflammation, inflammatory mediators and aging. NIA, Sept, 1-2, 2004).

Cellular damage by oxygen free radicals that results from the reactive oxygen species group of compounds used in inflammatory processes is a primary driving force for aging.

These oxygen free compounds also increase activation of redox-regulated transcription factors, which regulate the function of pro-inflammatory molecules that are seen in older animals and individuals, as opposed to their younger counterparts (all this is just scientific lingo for how inflammation plays a role in the aging process).

Hence, the reason why there is increasing use of anti-oxidant related vitamins and products. There are also increasing recommendations for consuming natural, less processed produce, as well as diets that are high in natural anti-oxidant minerals and substances.

There is an enzyme produced by the tissues of the body known human polynucleotide phosphorylase (hPNPaseold-35), which has been shown to be turned up or amplified during cellular division. This may represent a molecular link between aging and the associated age related inflammation. This substance also promotes reactive oxygen species production, and initiates the production of pro-inflammatory cytokines, such as IL-6 and IL-8 (Molecular mechanisms of aging-associated inflammation. Cancer Letters, Vol. 236, Issue 1, pgs. 13-23 (8 May 2006).

Based on the multiple articles published that I reviewed, there seems to be a preponderance of evidence that support the role of inflammation as a cause of aging. We are, however, far from identifying inflammation as the sole cause.

citizens categorized as obese (CDC://www.cdc.gov/obesity/data/trends.html).

Obesity is a product of multiple factors that can be categorized as inherited or acquired. By far, the majority of those who are overweight or obese belong to the acquired category. This is due to environmental influences. Most commonly, it is due to the fact that we consume more calories than we burn.

Many of the low-cost food items that make up fast foods contain high amounts of sugars and saturated fats, which are both high in calories. Added to this are the increasing portion sizes that have doubled since the 1970's. We can now begin to understand how and why our caloric intake has increased.

In 2000, Americans consumed an average of 57 more pounds of meat than they did annually in the 1950s. Furthermore, between 1950-1959 and 2000, the average consumption of added fats increased by two-thirds (USDA's Economic Research Service).

Americas' per capita consumption of sweeteners derived from cane, beet and corn also increased by a whopping 39% between 1950's and 2000.

By 2000, each American was consuming, on average, 152 lbs of sweeteners a year (USDA's Economic Research Service).

mation is associated
s and cardiovascular
seases have with

ch acid is not the
lcer disease, which
medical school and
called Helicobacter
consists of a multi-drug
biotic.

Chlamydia
the formation of arterial
rm during the process
arteries".

hronic inflammation,
ad to a wide range of

tious agents,
irus may also be causes
ions can be detected by

on, infectious diseases
cause of the majority of

Most of the illnesses and deaths that occurred i[n]
of the 20th century were caused by infections, m[any]
can now be easily treated with antibiotics.

This exposure to infectious material in our ance[stral]
may have caused the biology of our immune syst[em]
become highly active and responsive, which is w[hy]
such a crucial role in inflammation today. It may[ ]
why some individuals are more susceptible to m[ore]
episodes of particular illnesses.

In addition to the aforementioned causes of chro[nic]
inflammation, other factors such as cigarette sm[oking]
and the consumption of a pro-inflammatory diet
6, (like we have been consuming for decades), al[so]
to inflammation.

as obesity-related illnesses, is the number
[ ]ted issue affecting people in developed and
[cou]ntries alike.

[defin]ed as a body mass index (BMI) greater than
[ ]mass index is obtained from the persons'
[hei]ght. BMI, however, is not an ideal or accurate fat
[ ]it does provide a generalized idea of the person'[s]

[t]he 2007-2008 National Health and Nutrition
[S]urvey, obesity now affects 17% of all children
[and adolescen]ts in the United States—three times the rate of
[one g]eneration.

[ ] of adults in the U.S. were also considered obese[.]
[compar]ed to whites, blacks had a 51% higher rate of
[and H]ispanics had a 21% higher rate.

[ ]the 50 states had more than 20% of all their
[in th]e obese category—Washington D.C. and Colora[do]
[the onl]y two states with less than a fifth of all their

These are just some of the amazing facts and figures that give us an indication as to why we have become a fatter nation.

Obesity and Cancer

Although most of us know that obesity can cause diabetes and heart disease, most of us are unaware that obesity is also related to various types of cancer. The American Institute for Cancer Research reported convincing evidence which showed that the higher the percentage of body fat, the greater the risks for colorectal, esophageal, endometrial, pancreas, kidney, and breast cancer (WCRF/AICR. Food, Nutrition, Physical Activity and the Prevention of Cancer: a Global Perspective. World Cancer Research Fund/ American Institute for Cancer Research. 2007).

Possible mechanisms by which obesity can contribute to the development of cancer include: increased circulating levels of hormones, (which may increase risk for hormone-driven cancers), and decreased physical activity, which in turn can result in longer exposures to ingested toxins and chronic low-level inflammation (Visscher TL, Seidell JC. The public health impact of obesity. Annual review of public health 22355-75 2001).

Obesogens: Another Identifiable Cause of Obesity.

Another relatively new concept that is gaining acceptance as a contributor to the obesity epidemic, especially in young people, is the concept of obesogens.

By definition, obesogens are foreign compounds or chemicals that is thought to interfere with the metabolism of lipids, resulting in obesity.

In 2002, a medical researcher named Dr. Paula Baille-Hamilton published her work, which found that in the previous 40 years, obesity levels had increased in parallel to the increased use of pesticides and chemicals used in the plastics manufacturing industry. She was one of the first scientific researchers to identify a possible link between exposure to environmental toxins and obesity.

Other research followed that postulated a relationship between maternal exposure to these environmental toxins by the mother, with the effects on the fetus developing inside the uterus. This included newborns having a higher predisposition to becoming obese during the first months of life.

It has long been known that the intake of certain substances and medications by pregnant women could have negative effects on the development of the fetus and cause potentially damaging effects. This was the case with pregnant women that took the anti-nausea medication, Thalidomide, during the late 1950's. Unfortunately, the ingestion of this medication by the mother while pregnant, resulted in severe birth defects in many newborns. So the concept that exposure to some toxic substances or chemicals by the mother during pregnancy could then produce or be associated with changes in the offspring was already well established.

A review published in 2006 by the Harvard School of Public Health found a 74% increase in the numbers of overweight infants under 6 months of age, when compared to statistics of the previous 20 year period, starting in 1980 (Juhee Kim et.al "Trends in Overweight from 1980 through 2001 among Preschool-Aged Children Enrolled in a Health Maintenance Organization* Obesity (2006) 14, 1107-1112).

This finding of overweight and obese infants was quite unexpected, as it is impossible for infants under 6 months old to gain weight and become obese solely as a result of diet and caloric overconsumption.

which acts as an endocrine disruptor. Like Bisophenol A, under certain conditions and stimuli, tributyltin allows the cells to develop into fibroblasts and connective tissue. Under other stimuli, it can cause the precursor cells to development into fat cells.

Interestingly enough, activation of PPAR gamma by the diabetes medication, Avandia ™ and Actos ™ was the mechanism by which those drugs produced increased weight gain as a side effect.

Besides these two compounds, (Bisophenol A and tributylin), other chemicals have also been found that may cause endocrine dysregulation. These include phthalates used to make rolls of plastic food wrap, as well as perfluoroalkyl compounds, a substance that makes up the chemical compounds used and applied to the surface of the cooking pans to prevent food from sticking to them.

In a 2005 Spanish scientific paper, scientists demonstrated that the more pesticides a developing fetus is exposed to, the higher their risk of becoming overweight as children.

In 2008, scientists in Belgium, reported that fetuses exposed to high levels of pesticide such as DDT before their birth, become more overweight than those fetuses exposed to low levels.

Again, the amount of fat cells that form during intra-uterine development in the exposed fetus, will then remain with the individual for the rest of their life.

Recent research has also concluded that the obesogen stimulation can re-program the entire metabolic system, which pre-disposes the individual to becoming overweight or obese.

Another consequence of an increased number of adipocytes is that, in addition to being a store of fat, these cells also function in the regulation of the appetite. <u>Fat cells produce hormones that stimulate the brain to make us feel hungry. The more fat cells we have, the hungrier we feel and the more we eat.</u>

All these studies suggest a possible link between exposure to environmental toxins and chemicals during intra-uterine development and obesity.

A quick clarification: weight gain with aging, in people who have always been thin or of normal weight for most of their life, occurs because of poor dietary and lifestyle choices, and not because of obseogenes.

To reduce exposure to obesogens, you should limit the use of plastic containers that can leach out minute traces of these chemicals, especially when heated in microwaves. Rather than use these types of containers, you can store or keep your food in paper plates, aluminum foil or wax paper, or glass containers. If you still want to use plastic containers, before purchasing these, review the packaging labels. They should indicate whether or not the product is free of potentially toxic substances such as phthalates. Some of the newer plastic materials are being made without these chemicals, and state "BPA-free" (bisophenol A), directly on the container. Remember that many disposable plastic containers, such as those used for storage of water, oil, vinegar and other liquid food-stuffs, are also made from derivatives of these chemicals.

In a recently published study, researchers found that most of the plastic products tested, even some that claimed to be BPA-free, leached out these endocrine disrupting obesogens. Of the 455 plastic products examined, 70% had positive estrogen activity (Yang CZ, Yaniger SI, Jordan VC, Klein DJ, Bittner GD 2011. Most Plastic Products Release Estrogenic Chemicals: A Potential Health Problem That Can Be Solved. Environ Health Perspect. 03.02.2011).

Pre-natal pesticide exposure has now been demonstrated to be associated with a reduced IQ.

Organo-phospahates (used in pesticides) have recently been shown to decrease IQ levels in children that consume foods that contain traces of the pesticide. Research conducted by the Berkeley School of Public Health found that prenatal exposure to organophosphate pesticides, which is commonly used on crops, was associated lower intelligence scores at age 7. This study will soon be published in "Environmental Health Perspectives".

56

In addition, two additional studies conducted by Mt. Sinai Medical Center and Columbia Medical Center, also found similar associations between prenatal pesticide exposure and offspring affliction.

Taking Obese Kids Away From Their Families.

An article by researchers from Harvard University made headlines in July of 2011 when they suggested that child welfare agencies should be authorized to remove severely obese kids away from their families.

I disagree.

In the small amount of cases of such extreme child obesity, we need to recognize the possibility of obesogenes playing a role and contributing to cause the particular child's weight issue.

As physicians, we must be careful and explore all the possibilities in each individual case and not rush to drastic, "one size fits all" medical judgments and treatments. Unfortunately, a commonplace occurrence in how we practice medicine in America today. While protecting a child's health is everyone's responsibility, I am concerned that good parents may face expensive legal persecution and witch-hunts for something that is out of their control. It reminded me of parents wrongfully accused of child abuse based on incidental findings on x-rays of bony fractures in various stages of healing. Only after both the parents and their children were traumatized by forced separation, was the correct diagnosis of ostegenic imperfecta or brittle bone disease, caused by a genetic disorder made, rather than parental abuse or neglect.

In my opinion, the government need not be involved in the parenting business. They should instead provide incentives, education and more affordable healthy food choices, not threats or punishment.

Instead of recommending government intervention, these Harvard scholars, should have addressed the main causes of obesity, which are poor nutrition and lack of exercise.

Government would better serve us, the people, by helping subsidize production more of whole foods, lowering the cost of healthier foods and mandating physical education and nutrition classes in schools. Instead, we get Congress, going against U.S.D.A. recommendations and allowed pizza to be considered a vegetable, for school lunches!

It is sad to recognize how politicians can be so easily influenced. And while politicians continuously pass illogical laws that serve only a few, our country becomes fatter, sicker and healthcare costs continue to rise.

How fat tissue causes inflammation

Our body's fatty tissue, also known as adipose tissue acts like a functioning organ, as it can synthesize over 100 chemical substances that modulate body systems and functions. Furthermore, they secrete hormones that help regulate the immune system. These chemicals include pro-inflammatory substances called cytokines, which have multiple effects, including the up regulation of inflammation. (A good article on how adiposity causes cytokine production can be found in the journal, "Nature Medicine-12", 1359-1361 (2006).

In addition to cytokines, several other hormones are produced from fat, which play a crucial role in our metabolism. It wasn't until 1995, with the discovery that one of these fatty tissue produced hormones called leptin, that fat tissue was recognized as an endocrine organ.

Hormones that originate from fat include leptin, resistin and adinopectin. Currently, all of these three hormones are undergoing studies and research, as they may be modifiable causes that lead to obesity. Insulin, and leptin are the only two substances that have been identified to function as an adiposity signal or fat regulator.

Leptin circulates in proportion to body fat content, and has an important role in helping decrease and control our appetite. The more body fat one has, the higher the levels of circulating leptin. Leptin helps control our food intake by acting on receptors in the hypothalamus region of the brain. They act as a signal, indicating the degree of adiposity in the body, in a feedback loop type pattern.

In obese individuals, leptin levels are elevated, which can results in leptin resistance—much like the insulin resistance seen in individuals with metabolic syndrome and type 2 diabetics (N Engl J Med 334 (5): 292-295).

Leptin helps the growth of blood vessels by increasing levels of vascular endothelial growth factor. It also regulates the immune response to the atherosclerosis process, which is another possible mechanism for the increased atherosclerosis rate seen in obese patients (Arterioscler Thromb Vasc Biol. 27 (12): 2691-8).

Resistin, was discovered in 2001 and is associated with insulin resistance, hence the name "resistin". Increased resistin levels, are seen in obese individulas, as well as those with increased fat stores (J. Clin. Endocrinol. Metab. 88 (11): 5452-5).

Resistin has been linked to inflammation, as well as various other inflammatory processes (Obes. Res. 12 (6): 962-71),(EMBO J. 19 (15): 4046-55), (Transplant. Proc. 38 (10): 3434-6).

Remember again that chronic, low grade, persistent inflammation is bad and it is what we want to limit by way of nutrition, diet and lifestyle choices.

It is now believed that restistin plays a role and is involved in the association between obesity, insulin resistance, and chronic inflammation.

Circulating resistin levels were decreased, by the once popular anti-diabetic drug rosiglitazone (Avandia®), and are increased in diet-induced and genetic forms of obesity.

It is the fat located around our bellies and waist area that is called central adiposity. This fat contains the highest concentration of resistin, and it is this location, or content of fat cells, that is most related to insulin resistance and type 2 diabetes (J. Clin. Endocrinol. Metab. 88 (12): 6098-106), (Nature 409 (6818): 307-12).

Adenopectin is a hormone that regulates glucose regulation and fatty acid metabolism.

Like the other adipose derived hormones, adinopectin plays a role in insulin response. It also has anti-inflammatory effects on the endothelium, and it serves a protective function.

Levels of adinopectin are inversely related to adipose (fat) tissue and body fat. This means that the lower the levels of adinopectin, the more obese the individual may be.

High adenopectin levels (as seen with leaner individuals) are associated with decreased cardiovascular risks.

Adenopectin plays a role in obesity and in the development of atherosclerosis (Eur. J. Endocrinol. 148 (3): 293-300.), type 2 diabetes (J. Mol. Med. 80 (11): 696-702) and metabolic syndrome.

All of these fat derived hormones work in concert like a system of checks and balances—each one trying to maintain fat under control.

Fatter individuals should have a higher level of circulating leptin, in order to control and suppress hunger, which could result in reducing overall fat levels. However, as many overweight individuals have a simultaneous state of chronic low-level inflammation, resistance to leptin is common. This results in obesity. In addition, remember that adipose tissue is a rich source of cytokines (pro-inflammatory substances) that promote inflammation. Because of these influences, obesity can frequently cause continued inflammation and a cycle of chronic disease.

The state of our nations health and some healthcare statistics.

Healthcare has been, is and will always be, an important issue that is affecting us all, whether we realize it or not.

It does not matter how old you are or the state of your health at present. Whether you are a teenager flipping burgers part time for some spending money, or a 9 to 5 salaried worker, we are all impacted by, and have a stake in our country's escalating healthcare costs.

If you think about it, healthcare is the only issue that will affect and impact all of us at some point in our lives.

It is the central issue that will make us or break us, whether individually or as a country. Healthcare doesn't care if you are a Republican or Democrat, liberal or conservative, independent or indifferent. Healthcare is all of us people and should not be about the politicians or special interests in Washington that control it.

Consider America's healthcare as a ship that's loaded and bogged down. We are all in the same ship together, headed somewhere (somewhere because, with so many special interests vying for control, no one knows for sure where we are headed). If it is in a financially healthy state and we are all going in the same direction, it will be smooth sailing and we all benefit from it.

If, however, healthcare continues to struggle and we continue to fight ourselves over who is more right based on politics, the ship will go down and we all collectively go down with it. Lifeboats won't be able to save us from the catastrophic economic events that have the potential to occur if we continue on the current course.

That is why we all need to understand and care about the nations' escalating healthcare costs. These increasing costs continue to take a bigger slice of our economy as a result of multiple causes (although at a slower pace).

Some of these increased causes include: newer, more expensive technologies and medications that have resulted in the ability of sick individuals to live longer, the prolonging of life (and in many cases the prolonging of death), and from the curing and controlling of terminal medical conditions that were previously incurable. Illogical and incomprehensible health related legislation passed by politicians, who spend more time fund raising to stay in power, than actually working to help run a country.

Added to this is the "do more" mentality, which has been so commonplace in medical practice. A do more mentality fueled in part by the potential for additional monetary gains some physicians make, as defensive medicine to protect oneself from frivolous medical malpractice claims, and more commonly and important, the belief and expectations many patients have, that they are entitled to everything that medical technology has to offer, regardless of price or need.

No Medicare recipient, or a family member of a Medicare recipient, has ever asked me how much a test, procedure or therapy costs during my 16 years of practice.

This is especially true for the very debilitated, old, or chronically sick patients who have multi-system involvement and failure, and who are in critical condition in intensive care units on life support with no chance of survival. Many of whom have family members who despite being informed as to the seriousness and extremely poor prognosis, insist on everything being done medically to keep the patient alive. This includes, the continuation of futile, expensive care, which only serves in prolonging death.

Since they don't have to pay the bill, (you and I do, and our kids and grand kids will have to, as well), why would anyone bother to consider the costs and limited resources involved in prolonging death of their loved one, if even for a day?

America's increasing healthcare expenditures.

With each passing year, our nations population grows older. Many of those reaching older ages are suffering more from chronic illnesses, many of which result after a lifetime of poor lifestyle choices.

In 2011 alone, 7000 people a day, turned 65, and became eligible to receive Medicare benefits, for a total of 2.5 million additional beneficiaries added to Medicare in 2011 alone. The elderly are entitled to medical care, but the increase in numbers of beneficiaries contributes to increased health care costs.

(The Medicare program, is a Federal "entitlement" program, which started during the 1965 Johnson administration, in order to help cover medical costs of individuals 65 years of age or older. Later additions were made to include coverage for renal failure patients at any age, as well as a few other conditions).

The increased threat of malpractice lawsuits plays a role in the practice of defensive medicine. Defensive medicine leads to the ordering of additional tests, out of precaution rather than need, which adds to the overall U.S. healthcare expenditure.

Occasionally, some physicians may order diagnostic tests, not so much because it is truly needed, but rather as an added source of income. Although this is a small source of the additional increased healthcare costs, to be fair, complete and remain impartial, it is mentioned.

Lastly, healthcare costs are out of control, because we have no cohesive healthcare policy nor do we have the political will or leadership when it comes to establishing an equitable solution to this crisis. This means that both Democrats and Republicans will continue to side step the issue instead of coming up with an acceptable bipartisan solution. Failure to find a solution that reduces costs, while putting the health care needs of the people first, has the potential of leading our Country to its most serious and damaging economic collapse, which would be more catastrophic than the financial collapse of 2008.

There will probably be shared pain and hardship at some level fairly soon. (This manuscript was written before the debt ceiling crisis of July 2011, a crisis due in large part to escalating healthcare costs).

In 1980, Medicare expenditures was $34 billion, or 6% of total federal spending (TFS) of that year.

In 1990, Medicare expenditure was $107 billion (9% TFS), in 2000-$216 billion (12% TFS), in 2002-$257 billion (13% TFS), in 2004-$300 billion (13% TFS), in 2007-$435 billion (16% TFS), and in 2008-$600 billion (20% TFS).

In 2006, the Medicare prescription drug plan took effect to help with the cost of some common medications, which added another $49 billion to the total Medicare expenditures in 2008 alone.

Remember that these figures are of Medicare healthcare spending only.

Of the total healthcare costs, the payment breakdown for the U.S. population is as follows: 35% of the payments for healthcare services comes from private insurance, 34% from the federal government (in the form of Medicare), 13% from the states (Medicaid and others), 12% from our own out-of-pocket payment, and the remainder from other sources (U.S. Dept. of Health and Human Services, 2009a, "Personal Health Care).

When you add up all the payment sources that cover and are responsible for paying all our medical expenses, the total final annual healthcare expenditure is even higher.

Let's look again at the cost of Medicare in 2002. It was $257 billion dollars and represented only 34% of the total healthcare bill of that year. If we add to this amount, all the other amounts paid out by all the sources responsible in paying the nations healthcare bill that year, the total expenditure on healthcare in 2002 comes out to over $2 trillion dollars, that's a 2 followed by 12, 0's, $2,000,000,000,000.00!

We live in a fast paced world. Many families rely on the income of both working parents. Many, live their homes before the sun rises to beat traffic, drive hours to and from work each day, and get back home after the sun has set. We have homework, meetings, delays, pagers, cell phones, smart phones and other communication devices to contend with. Our kids have become latch key kids, locking themselves at home after school and passing the day by playing video games, working on the computer, surfing the internet, listing and downloading music and playing with ipods, and other electronic devices with little or no physical activity.

Add to these scenarios premade-packaged foods, fast foods, saturated fats, trans fats, high fructose corn syrup, sugar, soda, sweets, microwavable refined foods, junk foods and other processed foods. Foods, that are ready to eat, and that contain food additives, chemical food preservatives, artificial colorings and artificial flavorings.

Take all of the above factors, shake them well, add a sedentary lifestyle and presto! We have a nation of stressed out, unhealthy adults, and more importantly, stressed out, overweight and obese children, who until recently had the sad distinction of being the first generation in several decades to have a shorter life span than previous generations (A Potential Decline in Life Expectancy in the United States in the 21st Century," The New England Journal of Medicine 352, no. 11 (2005): 1138-45).

In addition to increased numbers of obese kids, adults who are suffering from increased rates of obesity, obesity related diseases as well as chronic inflammatory conditions that includes many of the most costly to treat, such as diabetes, cardiovascular diseases, pulmonary diseases, dementia, depression and cancer.

<u>Obesity has consistently been associated with almost all types of cancer,</u> many of which that are unfortunately on the rise—such as breast and prostate cancer (Calle EE, Rodriguez et al Overweight, obesity and mortality form cancer. NEJM 2003; 348:1625-1638).

<u>The United States is the country with the distinction of having the highest per capita expenditure on healthcare each consecutive year since 1980, with an average of $6102.00 per person in 2004</u> (www.cdc.gov).

This is a quick snap shot of our countries health in the 21st century, and it isn't a pretty picture.

Despite being the country that spends the most on healthcare, when we compare our infant mortality rate with 30 other countries, we find ourselves in an undesirably and high 3rd place. We have 6.9 infant deaths per 1000 live births, trailing only Mexico and Turkey who have higher infant death rates (OECD Health Data, 10/2006. CRS Report for Congress US healthcare spending: comparison with other countries. Sept 17, 2007 CRS-54).

When it comes to life expectancy at birth, of the top 50 countries in 2009, the United States was towards the bottom at number 48, with a slightly higher life expectancy than Guam and Albania (CIA world fact book 01/2009).

Forty-seven other countries had a higher life expectancy than Americans, and this does not yet reflect the anticipated decrease in life expectancy associated with the current generation of youths.

We need to ask ourselves, "What are we doing that leads us to have such poor outcomes? What is going on????

The statistics are frightening, but they are in plain black and white. Currently, in the United States, 65% of adults are considered obese and 16% of children and adolescents are overweight or obese. Another 15% of these are at risk of becoming obese (USA today 3/15/05).

<u>Childhood obesity levels have increased by a staggering 300%, when compared with levels from the 1970's.</u> Unfortunately, these levels continue to rise.

While our lives have become busier and more complicated, the time we devote to food selection, preparation and cooking, has decreased considerably or is non-existent. Consequently, we choose convenience, ready-made foods and are consuming more calories than ever before.

More and more, we are eating foods that contain a myriad of chemicals and substances that have been deemed and considered safe for human consumption. Chemicals and substances however, whose long-term health effects after chronic long-term consumption, have not been well established.

In addition to the increase in processed, refined, and high caloric foods, we have been consuming larger quantity of sugars, foods fried in fats (especially saturated and trans fats), and foods that contain disproportionately larger amounts of omega 6 fatty acids at the expense of the healthy omega 3 fatty acids.

We are also consuming larger servings and portions of foods. <u>Over the last 3 decades the size of food portions has in many cases doubled.</u> With it, so has the amounts of calories we consume. Since increased portion size has occurred gradually, many of us may not have been aware of this trend, while many more of us simply believe that larger food portions are a good value. We fail to realize the potential health risks associated with continuous, lifelong consumption of this kind. Large quantities of inexpensive, cheap foods have distorted our concept of what normal food portions should be. For your review, you are welcomed to check out a portion comparison quiz from the National Heart, Lung and Blood Institute website: (http://hp2010.nhlbihin.net/portion/index.htm).

In addition of going through our days eating foods of poor nutritional value, we have decreased the amount of exercise and physical activity we do. Because of financial issues, and monetary cutbacks, there are fewer school systems that offer physical education courses for our children. Furthermore, for many working families, it is safer for their kids to stay locked indoors at home after school, where they then remain sedentary. Adult activity habits and patterns are even worse than those of their children, because their hectic daily schedules makes setting time aside for exercise and taking care of oneself, a luxury many simply can't afford.

In addition to busy lives, we have just become a lazy people.

Over the last several years, I have seen an increase in the number of patients using motorized wheel chairs and medical scooters. Even at the local grocery store, people walk in, but apparently find it more convenient and easier to hop on a cart and drive around the store instead of walking. What makes me angry is the fact that many of the people I see riding around on these scooters are overweight and the ones that need to get off their butts and walk!

While patients with neurological or degenerative arthritic conditions certainly need and benefit from these mobility aids, the great majority of the people who use them would benefit more by walking with the assistance of a cane or walker.

What is worse is that Medicare pays for these motorized mobility devices in some cases, so it is we the people, who are subsidizing and helping pay for these expensive devices, some of which can cost up to $7000. It is no wonder why we have become an overweight, and unhealthy nation, and why we are all paying more for healthcare.

Inactivity and our sedentary lifestyles, especially among our youth, is another important factor that needs to be addressed in accordance with an anti-inflammatory diet and lifestyle. Weight loss obtained by exercise can prevent, reverse and/or delay heart disease, including cardiomyopathies, congestive heart failure, arterial disease, heart attacks, cholesterol and lipid abnormalities, and high blood pressure, metabolic syndrome, diabetes, sleep apnea, osteoporosis, depression, mental health, Alzheimer's, fibromyalgia, arthritis and many, many more. Exercise and physical activities are natural remedies—remedies which I consider more important than any prescription drugs. Anyone can do it at any time and place, free of charge and free of side effects.

Exercise is the best kept secret, as no one can bottle it and sell it by prescription!

As a cardiologist, I typically encourage at least 20 minutes of continuous, non-stop exercise 5 days a week. This minimal amount of physical activity promotes heart healthy effects. If a patient can walk into my office, we can find an exercise suitable for them to do, regardless of age. Although the more strenuous or intense the exercise, the more benefit obtained, physical activity does not need to be a grueling workout to be of benefit. Some patients simply cannot carry out intense physical activity.

In these cases, low intensity activity such as walking, household chores, gardening, or even recreational and work related activities can also help improve health.

Tai chi, a low impact martial arts type of exercise based on body movement, has been shown to improve all around mobility, health and wellbeing. It has been practiced for thousands of years and continues to be practiced today in many Asian countries, as well as in Asian communities across America, by older, wiser and more fit members of the community. Regardless of what activity you choose to start with, what is important is that you perform the activity continuously and consistently. More importantly, I would encourage the many who think they can't exercise, to start believing you can and at least give it a try.

Newton's first law of motion states that a body in motion stays in motion, while a body at rest stays at rest. This finding can be applied to our activities of daily living. I equate motion to life and being sedentary to death.

In addition to staying physically active and smoking cessation, recognizing and controlling stress and anxiety are important controllable factors that need to also be addressed in order to fully improve our health.

A nutritional walk down the last decades.

During the Second World War, while our troops where bravely fighting for our country abroad, many people here in the United States were involved in the agricultural and food industry. We needed to work to feed not just our troops and our own citizens, but many of the populations across Europe as well. These populations were facing rationings and severe food shortages as a result of the destruction of their agricultural infrastructure.

Because this country's demand for food products increased, the amount of food that needed to be produced similarly increased. In the United States, the government encouraged all its citizens to plant home gardens and grow their own fruits and vegetables in order to supplement their own personal food needs. This would also help decrease dependence on national food supplies. These so-called "Victory" gardens became a common sight throughout America—they could even be found on school and church grounds. A poll conducted in 1943, showed that 75% of Americans still processed and canned their own food at home (http://extension.usu.edu/aitc/lessons/pdf/ cc1940_war.pdf)

Americans were also soon required to accept rations of food and other commodities, including energy.

All across the country nutrition committees were being established to monitoring and utilize all available foods more efficiently in an effort to reduce food waste.

Industrial food preservation at that time consisted of canning, freezing, drying, and storing.

Individual farms and independent farmers still made up the backbone of our nations food system. In the 1940's, the number of acres that were farmed increased from 300,300 acres to over 536,900 acres. Similarly, the number of beef cattle, milk cows, and sheep also increased, as a result of increased livestock production.

Because of the larger amounts of food products that was being produced, newer methods for the preservation of food had to be developed. This was especially important and an urgent matter as the majority of the food was destined to be shipped tens of thousands of miles overseas.

At this time, unfortunately, we had inadequate preservation techniques, which consisted mainly of at home pickling, smoking, and dehydration, in addition to the previously mentioned commercial techniques of canning, freeze drying and flash freezing. The lack of any widely available, reliable refrigeration systems, added to the inadequate commercial preservation techniques of the time.

After the war, the food preserving and additive industry began to grow. This was a result of the technology acquired during the war, which gave rise to frozen foods and TV dinners, as well as the start of the processed foods and the snack industry—all of which are produced with large amounts of chemical preservatives.

Large-scale food production began to be led by several corporations, which would in a short period of time revolutionize the agriculture-food industry. Industrial farming comprising of thousands of acres of crops would require not only newer fertilizers and pesticides to increase yield, but increased automation and technology as well. Mechanization quickly improved and was relied on to handle the increasing production volumes, as well as to compensate for the severity of the labor shortages of that time.

Towards the end of the 1940 's, the McDonald's brothers in California began to introduce a new food vending system that would revolutionize the way we eat. A system of selling meals which later would become known as fast food—a concept in which a smaller selection of food items could be prepared and served quickly. Typically, these foods were prepared from pre-cooked food components on an assembly line.

After World War II, an era of prosperity began in America. Soldiers returned home, married, started families, and settled across all parts of the country, extending the population from coast to coast. This expansion was made possible by the construction of hydroelectric dams in the West, as well as the Interstate Highway Act of 1956, which would led to the establishment of the country's interstate highway system. The infrastructure necessary to facilitate transportation of goods and services across the entire nation was thus created.

The end of the 1950's and the beginning of the 1960's brought with it road expansions that could take us to locations and places that had been previously inaccessible and isolated. Accordingly, there was a tremendous increase in the number of motor vehicles sold, including motorcycles.

We were a nation on the go, enjoying our hard earned freedom and stature in the world, which came after years of sacrifice.

Another factor that forever would change the way we eat and our system of nutrition was the expanding McDonald establishments. Expansion that became possible through the development of the franchise model.

Fast food type of meals became successful because the food tasted good, was filling, inexpensive, and quick. As a result, this type of food establishment caught on quickly. Within a short period of time, other fast food franchises emerged and joined the McDonald's brand, in expanding rapidly across the United States.

As a result of these franchise restaurants, led by McDonald's, the basic food items to be used in their menus such as the beef, chicken, pork, potatoes, lettuce, and tomatoes, had to be purchased in ever increasing quantities. More importantly, these products needed to be of uniform consistency in order to be able to reproduce and obtain the same exact quality and flavors in all franchise outlets throughout the entire country.

This caused the need for standardization in the production of the farm animals as well as in the cultivation of the crops.

Producers and manufacturers of these products needed to adhere to the same guidelines in order to satisfy the increasing demands of items required by this newly flourishing type of business.

We were also entering the Cold War and the era of space exploration and the space race. The United States Air Force was expanding, NASA was born, and new scientific discoveries followed. New manmade compounds and materials were created, as were a variety of newer, synthetically produced chemicals that would allow the production of other substances. Plastics, nylon and other synthetic materials were developed from single molecules and basic molecular building blocks. Technologies in refrigeration, logistics, early computers all came into existence. Soon, a growing nation and other military wars and conflicts would require newer methods of food preservation.

In 1957, a newly developed orange-flavored drink powder was produced. This new form of drink, gained national recognition when it was included on the Gemini space flights. Tang®, was the name of that product, and it still exists today.

By applying newly acquired scientific discoveries, private sector corporations became increasingly involved and active, in the research and development of food. Modification of food into their basic components was made possible, which in turn led to the creation and formulation of new kinds of edible food items. Because of the intense research and development occurring in the field of food additives, the Food and Drug Administration (FDA), established the Foods Additives Amendment of 1958. This amendment introduced and set, minimal safety standards that are still in use today.

"Generally recognized as safe" is a common FDA designation applied to the chemical substances used in food product preparation, to designate them as being considered safe.

During the 1960's, we as individuals began to increase in weight. All of the factors needed for the start of our weight gain were in place, led by fast food and a decrease in our levels of physical activity.

As a result of our weight gain, artificial sweeteners and sugar substitutes were created as an alternative to sugar. These substances reproduce the taste of sugar with little or no calories, and were considered to be one of the first "diet" substances. Some of the most popular sugar substitutes included cyclamate (created in 1958 and later banned in 1970 due to its association with bladder cancer in rats), aspartame (1965), acesulfame-potassium and saccharin (1967), the latter three of which are still in use today.

In addition to the many artificial sweeteners created between 1965 and 1970, the industrial production of high fructose corn syrup (HFCS) was first established. It became possible to take corn, add some enzymes and chemicals, and with some changes to their chemistry, create a sugary tasting product. We will discuss HFCS later on.

The food preservation industry also flourished with the creation of chemical substances such as nitrates, sulfates, sodium bisulfate, starch, corn starch, artificial colors, artificial flavors, hydrogenated oils, potassium chloride, mono and diglycerides, soybean oil, monosodium glutamate, soy flour, lecithin, dipotassium phosphate and many others that are still used today in the food industry.

In addition to development of these chemical preservatives, food was also starting to be preserved and contained by a newly created substance known as "plastic". Plastic, would quickly replace the tin containers and glass bottles of the time.

Food production

In the 1970's, the five largest American companies involved in agricultural production controlled 25% of the agri-industry market. Science and technology continued making great strides, and new cultivation and animal raising techniques were developed.

To continue to increase efficiency, yield and output of these agricultural products, industrial farms where born. Farms grew from a few hundred acres (the typical size of independent farms of the 1940's) to farms thousands of acres in size. To be able to increase yield, chemical fertilizers and pesticides began to be increasingly employed. Increasing amounts of irrigation water was also needed, as was an increase in the level of mechanization. All of this required a large amount of capital investment. With continued advances in technology, farm machinery got bigger and more expensive. Tractors, combines and other farm equipment were using the latest technology and becoming state of the art. Farm machinery gradually being equipped with newer sensors, computers, GPS and other electronic systems that allowed them to practically run themselves. These machines cut down on harvest time, while increasing production yield. Crop rotation techniques, which allowed for more efficient and continued year—round farming across the country was also being employed. The positive end result of this type of large-scale farming was that the prices of crops and produce decreased, product availability increased and most importantly, consistency was continually be maintained, keeping with the needs of the franchise restaurants. These changes in industrial farming made it possible for a franchise-brand burger and fries purchased in Tampa to taste the same as one bought in Tupalo.

On the other hand, the inability of independent small farmers to come up with and raise the large investment of capital required to set up a large scale operation, in addition to their growing operating costs and decrease in revenues, made it difficult for the dwindling numbers of active individual farmers remaining, to be able to compete with the giant industrial agricultural corporations. After generations of farming, many independent farmers were forced to either sell to their larger competitors, or were forced out of business.

Today, those same 5 companies that controlled 25% of the agricultural and food production market in the 1970's, control 80% of the industry.

This consolidated control extends to include the sector responsible for the production of livestock and animals to be used for human consumption.

There is no doubt that the majority of us have been unaware and even ignorant as to how the meats and produce we consume in this country are produced, as well as who produces it.

Again, we are busy with our lives. The food we eat is the last of our many concerns. Many perhaps also believe that the government is actively looking out for our health and best interest, and never bother to think about the quality of the food we consume.

But just like the changes that occurred with the agricultural produce suppliers, who consolidated, decreased in numbers while increasing market share, so too did the needs of fast food franchise restaurants also change. They too demanded a more efficient economy of scale and a similar standardization when it came to the meat suppliers.

Centralization and product control began in response to the millions of tons of meat required per month by these worldwide fast food establishments. As a result, industrial sized farms that could contain thousands of variant animals (from cattle, to pigs, to turkeys) or any other large concentration of animals were created. These large farms became known as concentrated feeding operation or CAFO's.

The U.S. Environmental Protection Agency (EPA), describes a CAFO as "an agricultural operation where animals are kept and raised in confined areas. Facilities where these animals congregate, feed, manure and urinate on a small land area. Feed is brought to the animal rather than the animal grazing or seeking food in pastures, fields or on a range". Again this is the EPA definition.

Interestingly enough, the term CAFO as per the EPA, also describes facilities that pose potential pollution problems (www.epa.gov/cafo).

<u>Over 10 billion animals are consumed annually in the U.S. and 80% to 90% of these animals are chickens.</u>

In the United States, chicken has become the most consumed type of meat. On average, we consume 86 pounds a year per person, compared to 65 pounds each, for beef and pork (www. meatAMI.com). Daily, from 72,000-100,000 cattle are killed for meat (varies depending on the report quoted) and over 288,888 pigs and hogs are killed. That's each day (USDA Livestock Slaughter Summary, April 2011—http://usda01.library. cornell.edu/usda/current/LiveSlauSu/LiveSlauSu-04-25-2011.pdf).

(Remember, as previously mentioned, that we also consumed 152 lbs. of sweeteners per person, in 2002)!!

To be able to meet these increased meat demands, cattle and meat production as well as the way these animals are raised, changed forever.

Naturally bred chickens, traditionally required an average of 70 days from hatching to maturity to be processed. Like cattle and other farm animals used for human food consumption, chickens have traditionally fed on an assortment of grains, herbs and other natural nutrients found in the soil. They would graze outdoors exposed to the sun and fresh air, as well as to all of the nutrients and minerals found in the earth.

This is a far cry from the way in which chickens and other animals are bred and raised today, which is not only different, but tragically sad.

Instead of the traditional and natural, free—range, organic method of raising chickens, chickens are now raised similar to cattle, confined to CAFO's. Chickens are now raised in concentrated industrial farms, enclosed in structures that can contain hundreds and thousands of these animals.

They are typically kept in cages, or are grouped together with little or no space between them, in climate-controlled environments.

Many chickens are raised and kept in complete darkness, with no natural light and no natural fresh air. These animals mature quicker than their natural, normal growth, never seeing the light of day or being exposed to a normal environment. Instead they spend 24 hours a day confined to a small, crowded and restricted space where movement is limited.

You can only imagine what the sanitary conditions must be like in these hot and poorly ventilated industrial hen houses. Chickens raised in coops overwhelming with the stench of feces and waste by-products (which tend to smell of concentrated ammonia).

Because there are thousands of chickens at a time under these unsanitary yet acceptable conditions, antibiotics are routinely given to prevent bacterial over-growth and disease. These animals are not fed their traditional diets of natural grains, grasses, bugs, weeds and other natural components; rather they are fed scientifically manufactured compounds that contain corn, which will result in a fast weight gain that is also less expensive. <u>Instead of a traditional, normal growth period of 70 days, science and technology has sped up chicken growth to 45 days.</u> This amounts to a reduction of 37%, in the normal growth and development time. In my opinion, a reduction that parallels a 37% reduction in the quality of the meat produced, over traditionally raised chickens.

What has resulted is a "uniform", low cost product of limited variety, which nonetheless meets the standards required by the franchise and the food industry alike. An end product of the same consistency, size, composition, and flavor has thus been produced.

When McDonald's needed chickens with larger breast meat for use in their newly launched chicken product, a new breed of genetically modified chicken was developed, that was able to develop a larger sized breast meat of equal consistency.

As I mentioned previously, there are only 4 or 5 multinational corporations in the United States today that control the entire agricultural food industry. This includes the production of foods produced from livestock and other animals.

The largest U.S. supplier of chickens, as well as beef products, is credited with the creation of this new class of chicken. Currently, this same corporation provides its brand products to 88 of the 100 largest food franchise businesses.

Next time we eat a piece of chicken from any national franchise, notice the size of the chicken piece you are about to consume. You may undoubtedly notice that it is much larger than the size of a traditional chicken breast.

The raising of cattle, pigs and other animals for human consumption occur in a similar manner: being controlled by a few multinational corporations that supply meat product throughout the country. Remember that the number of agricultural-food producing companies in the United States has been steadily decreasing over time. The same corporation responsible for the creation of the new type of chicken with larger breast size incrementally acquired a total of 20 smaller competing food companies over the last 20 years. This establishes them as the largest producer and supplier of animal based foods.

When it comes to the production of beef and other meats, production of scale is also important to keep costs down. It is cheaper and more cost effective to run a production operation that deals in volume, as opposed to smaller operations. This is an economy of scale.

Pigs and hogs are omnivores, meaning they will eat just about anything, including both plants as well as other animal protein.

Cattle and dairy cows have traditionally been herbivores, consuming diets based on grasses and grains, which are rich in healthy omega 3 fatty acids.

Traditionally, these animals have been raised on large open spaces where they roam freely, eating a variety of natural grasses and grains that arise directly from fields and pastures, replete with natural vitamins, minerals and other beneficial nutrients. Being and moving around outdoors, exposed to the sun, having access to clean drinking water, as well as their natural, healthy diets, required a longer time for their growth and development, but made the beef lean and nutritious. Again, this in stark contrast to a CAFO, in which scientifically manufactured feed is brought to the animals.

In many CAFO's today, corn has become the ingredient of choice in animal feeds. Corn is abundant, making it a cheap ingredient. In addition, it is a high calorie grain, which is beneficial in fattening up the animals that consume it on a regular basis, including us humans. As I will later mention, corn is also used as a filler in many of the processed foods we consume today.

In addition to corn, soy is increasingly being used in animal feed. Both of these commodities are predominantly composed of omega 6 fatty acids, instead of the healthy omega 3 fatty acids typically found in natural grasses and grains, as well as in the meats of grass feed animals.

Humans need both of these essential fatty acids with slightly more omega 6 than omega 3. However, our traditional Western diet, consisting of processed and fast foods, is loaded with more of the omega 6 fatty acid. Consequently, we are consuming less omega 3 fatty acids, and increased amounts of omega 6, which contributes to the development of chronic inflammation and diseases.

I will delve into further discussion of these fatty acids in later coming chapters.

Animal feeds are abundant and cheap. They function in fattening up animals more quickly, decreasing the growth time, reducing production cost. As a result, the price we pay at the grocery store or restaurants is lower than the more traditionally farm raised beef products.

Technology has found ways to bring down the cost of beef and meat production, making them more affordable. As a result, consumption of meat in the United States has increased.

The end result of our nations meat production is a scientifically studied, refined and controlled growth and manufacturing process, which results in animal products of similar consistency and little variation.

In some European countries, in addition to grasses and grains that made up their feeds, soybean meal had been used as the principal plant based protein additive in their cattle feed. European countries would often have to import soybeans and other feed materials because their environmental and climatic conditions made the harvest and production of these grains impossible.

As the cost of soybeans increased, farmers had to find more affordable alternatives to substitute soy and other traditional feeds. Some European cattle growers began using protein from processed meat and bone meal components left over from ground and cooked processed waste products of slaughtered animals.

Leftover parts and remains of chickens, sheep and pigs, as well as the cadaveric remains and carcasses of sick and injured animals that would be milled, cooked, and added to feed as a protein supplement.

The use of this kind of protein meal, which was acceptable in Europe in the early to mid 1980's, was one of the main causes responsible for the outbreak of encephalitis in cattle that occurred in England at the end of the 1980s. This disease, known as bovine spongiform encephalopathy, was more commonly referred to as "Mad Cow Disease" and was responsible for over 200 deaths worldwide. This excluded the United States, where no cases occurred.

The United States Agriculture Department, (USDA) is responsible for ensuring the quality of our beef and meat supply. As is the case with many government agencies responsible for oversight and safety, the USDA has a limited amount of employees and resources. Often, they must rely on the word of the food industry they regulate, to assure that quality standards are being met. The health, safety and the interest of the American consumer are balanced with the interest of the industry.

In 2006, for example, the USDA prevented a Kansas beef producer from taking additional independent safety checks, to ensure that his meat products were safe from Mad Cow Disease. ("Mad cow watch goes blind". USA Today. 2006-08-03). http://www.usatoday.com/news/opinion/editorials/2006-08-03-our-view_x.htm).

Makes you wonder whose interest the USDA is really looking out for?

Changes in our food supply.
Cloning/Genetically Modified Foods

Cloning started to become a reality by 2001. From 2001 until 2008, the Food and Drug Administration (FDA) conducted studies on the safety of cloned foods destined for human consumption. In 2008, the FDA concluded that meats cloned from healthy cattle, swine and goats were as safe as non-cloned foods for humans to consume. They went ahead and gave permission for the sale of meats and milk from cloned cattle and cows, but the USDA intervened and asked producers to keep the sale of cloned products off the U.S. market. So far, the sale of these products remains nonexistent. Another point to take into consideration is that in the United States there is no law established, requiring the identification or labeling of meats and animal products, as originating from a cloned source.

Genetically modified organisms other than animal products have managed to find their way into our food supply, mainly in the form of seeds.

Genetically modified seeds, where marketed with the claim that these seeds where more resistant to different diseases, drought, and the chemical glycophosphate—the highest selling weed-killer on the market.

Genetically modified foods, or the genetically modified organisms (GMO), like seeds that produce them, first appeared on the U.S. market during the 1980's.

GMO's are protected by patent laws and intellectual property laws, making them the exclusive property of the corporations that created them.

The following common food items are grown from genetically modified seeds: 93% of the soybean crops, as well as 93% of the canola and cottonseed oil production, and 86% of our corn. Next year, genetically engineered rice will be introduced to the market place.

The use of genetically altered seeds is not exclusive to the United States. Brazil, Argentina and India follow the U.S. in volume of GMO produced food items. Some estimates have put the percentage of genetically modified food in the U.S. market at a staggering 75%. (www.gmaonline.org).

Vaccines.

Vaccines are administered to mature cattle and other animals in two ways.

The first vaccine administered to cattle is to prevent diseases and to help the animal stay healthy and survive until they are ready for slaughter.

The second vaccines is administered to mature cattle, in order to improve the survival of the animal, as well as to protect the unborn animal fetus and improve the reproductive status of the animal.

Antibiotics.

According to a 2001 article in Scientific American, <u>over seventy percent (70%) of all antibiotics manufactured in the United States annually, (about 25 million tons), are used in the agricultural sector and administered to livestock!</u> (Scientific American Jan 10, 2001).

I thought I was someone fairly knowledgeable and current on many health related statistics, but nothing could have prepared me for this astonishing number.

In fact, it was this particular statistic that made me start reading and researching as much as I could about our foods, causing me to pen what would eventually become this book. This fact alone should be a wake up call to all of us to the reality of the quality of the foods we eat.

Hormones.

In addition to antibiotics, synthetic bovine somatotropin hormone was first used on livestock in 1994.

Administration of this hormone to cows causes an increase in milk production of approximately 18 kilograms (39lbs.) per cow, per day. Increased milk output and production was reached at the expense of a 25% increase in the cases of utter mastitis and a 40% reduction in cow fertility.

Currently, 60% of the milk produced for human consumption in the United States is produced by cows that are treated with this synthetic hormone.

The U.S. is the only developed country that allows its citizens to drink milk from cows injected with hormones. Countries belonging to the European Union, as well as Australia, Canada, and various others prohibit its sale.

In September 2010, during a presentation to an appellate court in the U.S., it was shown that milk produced from cows that were treated with synthetic bovine growth hormone contained elevated levels of the hormone IGF-1 and higher levels of pus, which caused the milk to sour more quickly (www.grist.org / article / food).

Growth implants

Growth implants are synthetic hormones administered to nursing calves in order to increase their weight and speed up their growth by increasing the secretion of growth hormone and insulin.

There are three different types of estrogen implants. One consisting of a hormone combination of estradiol benzoate and progesterone, the other is composed of zeranol, and the last one consists of estradiol—all of which are synthetic hormones.

In 1997, only 14% of small producers (less than 300 cows) were using these substances but 55% of large producers (more than 300 cows), used it routinely (aces.nmsu.edu/pubs/_b/b-218.pdf).

All of these hormones, antibiotics, vaccines, and chemicals eventually enter the circulation of the animal and find their way into the tissues, including the meat in varying minute amounts, which individually have shown to produce no ill effect. It is thought, however, that with time and with chronic ingestion by humans, a cumulative effect may occur that triggers stimulation of our inflammatory and immune system. This consequently produces varying degrees of chronic inflammation that then may develop into chronic diseases.

Fruits, vegetables and many other crops use to have a typical growing season. But because of GMO's and agricultural advances and importation, we can obtain any fruit or vegetables throughout the entire length of the year, often at the expense of their nutritional composition and value.

Many large—scale commercial farming practices utilize man-made, compound fertilizers, composed mainly of phosphorus, nitrogen and oxygen molecules in order to sustain the nutritional requirements of the year-round crops. This is done at the expense of other assortments of natural elements and irreproducible trace minerals found in unadulterated soil. The repeated planting of the same seed type without crop rotation also causes a depletion of many of these natural soil minerals, resulting in crops that contain less vitamins and nutrients, and less of the natural anti-oxidant phytochemicals.

Many crops are harvested with fertilizers and pesticides and shipped with preservatives, allowing for their extended shelf life.

<u>As a result, many fruits and vegetables we buy today contain traces of pesticides and other chemical residues</u>.

These substances can be found on the leaves and stems, and they can penetrate the root of the plant, becoming part of the final product.

The Environmental Working Group (www.ewg.org), publishes an annual list of the most contaminated fruits and vegetables based on the levels of pesticides used in their cultivation.

According to their research, the most contaminated fruits in descending order are: peaches, apples, sweet peppers, celery, nectarines, strawberries, cherries, pears, grapes, imported spinach, and potatoes.

Foods that are grown with small amounts of pesticides include: papaya, broccoli, cabbage, banana, kiwi, frozen peas, asparagus, mango, pineapple, frozen corn, avocado and onion.

The regular use of fertilizers and pesticides creates another potential public health problem as approximately <u>70% of all of the fresh water available worldwide is used in the agricultural industry.</u> <u>The irrigation water run off becomes contaminated by agri-chemicals that then drains and pollutes the ground water and aquifers.</u> These are the sources of the drinking water for many of our largest cities.

Not only are we being exposed to chemicals and foreign substances in the food we are eating, but many of the natural sources of our drinking water are contaminated as well.

Our digestive tract and disease

We know that food is essential for our survival, but many are not aware that metabolizing and converting food into energy is taxing on our body. <u>Converting food into energy causes an increase in cellular stress, especially oxidative stress.</u> When consumption is intermittent and sporadic, this stress is beneficial. However, <u>when food consumption is excessive and continuous,</u> much like it is and has been in our lives, <u>it leads to DNA damage directly via oxidative pathways and indirectly via adipose related pro-inflammatory cytokine production.</u>

We need to remember that we, (our bodies and our physiology) came from and are descendants of hunter-gatherers—people who lived during times when food was scarce and we ate sporadically. When our days revolved around the finding and gathering of food to sustain us for the day. Although we have advanced and developed, much of our current constitutional make-up still dates back to those primitive characteristics.

Remember again that our trend towards becoming overweight, obese and suffering from increased rates of chronic illnesses started during the 1950's and 60's as previously described.

Before then, we ate sparingly, nutritiously and the majority of the population was lean.

Many of our current, common everyday foods are some of the many nutritional sources that can contribute to states of chronic inflammation, obesity, digestive disorders and other chronic diseases.

These foods contain antibiotics, hormones, growth factors, and vaccines as previously described and are packed with additives such as preservatives, coloring, flavoring and other chemicals.

Interestingly enough, many health conditions occasionally start out as non-specific digestive symptoms as a result of alterations and damage to the intestinal flora. This occurs with chronic ingestion of toxins, irritants, medications and food.

The intestinal flora

Before birth, our digestive tract is sterile and free of pathogen-causing bacteria. As we travel out through the birth canal during delivery, we begin to seed our digestive tract with our mothers bacterial micro-flora, acquired from the bacteria's found in the birth canal. Eventually our digestive tract is settled by thousands of different bacterial species all of which play an integral part of our digestive and immune system.

(I'd like to mention that babies born by way of a cesarean section have a disadvantage, as they do not acquire these important bacteria. Indeed, studies have shown that as a result, babies born via a C-section have a higher risk of respiratory allergies, asthma, celiac disease and allergies to milk products).

The human intestine usually contains an average of 100 to 200 trillion (100-200,000,000,000,000) microorganisms, consisting of viruses and bacteria referred to as the intestinal flora. Collectively, this is also known as the microbiome. Most of these microorganisms are good microbes functioning to keep us healthy by breaking down toxins and disease-producing pathogens.

Having a total weight of about 4 pounds, these microorganisms are essential and indispensable for our body's physiological processes, such as for the digestion of food, as well as normal digestive functioning. There is a similar bacterial flora located on the surface of the skin, but the most important one belongs to the digestive tract.

These bacteria are important in the prevention of illness and diseases, and helps in the regulation of inflammation within the digestive tract. Alterations or destruction of the normal digestive bacteria and microorganisms has been found to be the cause of a diverse range of systemic diseases ranging from irritable bowel syndrome to cystic fibrosis.

There is a growing amount of evidence that demonstrates a close relationship between inflammatory states and the immune system with the digestive tract, in the development of diseases. A relationship that includes playing a role in states of anxiety and depression. For example, people who suffer from inflammatory bowel disease (IBD) experience 3 times the rate of depression than those without IBD (Fuller, Thompson 2000, http:// onlinelibrary. wiley.com/doi/10.1097/00054725-200608000-00005/full).

Anxiety and depression affects as many as 60-80% of patients during exacerbations of IBD, causing a proposed link between these conditions (The hygiene hypothesis and psychiatric disorders G.A.rook Trends in Immunology April 2008 29(4):150-8).

Over the last several years there has also been increasing interest in the function of these digestive tract microbes in the reduction or increase of risk for disease, including colon cancer (Bosscher D. etal Food-based strategies to modulate the composition of the intestinal microbiota and their associated health effects. Journal of physiology and pharmacology :60 Suppl 65-11 Dec, 2009).

There is now growing evidence demonstrating the relationship between the digestive tract, the immune system and the brain. This is especially true of the relationship that exists between chronic digestive system inflammation with depression and anxiety states.

Adding to the growing evidence of the important health benefits of these intestinal bacteria is a recent study from Duke University. It indicated that an imbalance of the bacteria that make up our natural microbiome might also be responsible for some allergies, diabetes and obesity.

The biodiversity of the bacteria, viruses and microbes that make up our intestinal microbiome is necessary and responsible for maintaining our health and stimulating our immune system. It is not the cause of disease, as many had previously thought.

In other words, it is not the presence of these bacteria that cause disease, but rather it is their destruction and/or their damage that eventually leads to illness and disease.

One of the most common causes of damage to the beneficial microbes that make up our intestinal flora is the use of antibiotics.

The indiscriminate overuse of antibiotics has become a serious problem in our society, resulting in many adverse consequences. These include the emergence of drug resistant bacteria and an alteration of our digestive tract bacteria.

As a society, we are inappropriately taking too many antibiotics for the wrong reasons. We forget that these are powerful drugs that, in addition to killing disease-causing bacteria, also kill health promoting, good bacteria. Think of antibiotics like chemotherapy: it is a beneficial drug when used correctly for the right reasons, but one that will inadvertently kill everything in its path if inappropriately used. Besides the intentional overuse of antibiotics, many of us fail to take into account that the animals whose meat products we have consumed over the years, at some point have been treated with additives that include antibiotics. (Remember again, the Scientific American article on the use of antibiotics in the food industry). Even though the amount that may be found in our food supply is miniscule, its continuous consumption chronically over time can, by itself and in combination with other factors, eventually lead to damage of the bacteria and other microbes that make up the intestinal flora.

In addition to the inappropriate use of antibiotics, chronic stomach-acid suppressing medications can also lead to destruction of good digestive tract bacteria.

This is far too common, especially amongst the elderly who continuously take these drugs for months and even years at a time.

Although the indication for the use of these medications may have been appropriate at first—to suppress acid production in an attempt to relive acid reflux and heartburn—I commonly see patients taking them continuously, long after the recommended course of treatment.

Many continue to take these drugs, believing that if they stop, their digestive symptoms of abdominal bloating, pain and burning will return. They thus initiate a vicious cycle of chronic medication use.

What many may not be aware of is that the continuous use of these acid-suppressing medications may themselves become the cause of their continued, non-specific digestive symptoms.

Nonspecific digestive symptoms that include abdominal bloating, pain, burning, cramping, discomfort or heaviness, changes in bowel habits, nausea as well as many other symptoms, many of which are not typically associated with digestive issues. Symptoms that may include tiredness, loss of energy, irritability, body aches, fatigue and others

By decreasing and changing the pH and acidity of the stomach, acid-suppressing medications allows the growth of potentially harmful microorganisms which are responsible for the production of many of these non-specific symptoms.

In addition to producing these symptoms, the continuous use of acid suppressers has also been associated with hip fractures and pneumonia. The "proton pump inhibitor" class of acid suppressors has been associated with interfering with calcium absorption, which could contribute to osteoporosis.

Allergy to different types of foods is also becoming more recognized, whether it is from better awareness or a true increase in the number of sufferers. In the better awareness category, we have people that have allergies to food additives such as food colorings and dyes. This is being recognized more frequently in children. Currently, it is an area of increased scientific study with diverse findings, although no definite conclusions.

Other people naturally are allergic to products like soy, peanuts, wheat and/or corn.

An interesting finding, obtained from a recent study conducted by the University of Maryland, was one that showed that a large number of people who did not test positive for celiac disease (allergy to gluten—a protein component of wheat and barley) showed improved digestive symptoms when they went on a gluten free diet. The conclusion being that even in people who test negative on a screening, if symptoms continue and seem to be associated with a certain food or macronutrient, an elimination of the suspected food item should be tried. In cases such as these, patients were still considered gluten sensitive, despite a negative test result (http://somvweb.som.umaryland.edu/absolutenm/templates/?a=1474).

People can be gluten sensitive and have a normal screening test, but on eliminating wheat products they respond with rapid and marked improvements, as if they did have the illness.

The numbers of sufferers of gluten sensitivity has seemingly increased in numbers over the last several decades. In a retrospective study by the Mayo Clinic, stored blood samples of 10,000 Air Force reservists from the 1960's were analyzed. The findings revealed a four-fold increase in the incidence of gluten sensitivity today (http://www.mayoclinic.org/ news2009-rst/5329.html).

Again, no one knows for sure why this is happening but it seems that there is something triggering our immune system to attack the ingested gluten.

Another probable contributor to many of our digestive complaints and symptoms is stress.

Whether it is stress or an allergic response to any component of the nutrients we consume, the additives or chemicals used in the manufacturing, processing and preservation of food, our bodies can be impacted both beneficially or as is increasingly the case, negatively by what and how we eat.

Probiotics

An increased recognition and better understanding of the importance of the microbiome and function of digestive bacteria in maintaining our health, is part of the reason for the increase in sales of a class of supplements known as probiotics.

The definition of probiotics, according to World Health Organization is: "live micro-organisms, which when supplied in sufficient quantities, results in a salutary effect."

Probiotics were created in the 1980s, and are used to improve digestion. Specifically, to help restore and replenish the numbers of bacteria in the microbiome of the digestive tract that have been lost to a variety of causes, including the ones mentioned previously.

Probiotics are substances and compounds composed of millions of bacteria and enzyme products of these bacteria. They are taken orally in order to add and increase the number of good bacteria present in the digestive tract. Probiotics help improve digestive tract motility, regulation, and repair.

The most common bacterias utilized as probiotics include lactobacilli and bifidobacteria. Probiotic supplements come in capsule form, or they are incorporated and added to foods, such as soy or dairy products like milk and yogurt.

In my practice, when patients complain of non-specific digestive complaints, I review the medications they are currently taking and more importantly, the length of time they have been taking them.

I then discontinue medications (when appropriate) and recommend making small changes to the diet, as well as suggesting a trial of probiotics use. After several weeks, many feel relief and resolution of their abdominal discomfort. Others claim to feel better than they had in years. Sometimes, we have also been able to discontinue medications that had been taken indiscriminately for years.

I hope this section allows you some understanding of the importance of the digestive tract microbes, the quality of the food we eat and their role in our health and wellbeing.

The role of corn.

Some have proclaimed corn as the king of all crops because not only can be found in a large variety of foods and foodstuffs, but because it is also a component of a wide variety of non edible products as well.

Of all the grain crops produced in the United States, corn became the dominant and most abundant crop. This is partly as a result of government subsidies that started in 1995.

These subsidies were granted to producers of food grains, namely soybeans, wheat and corn. Most subsidies however, were given to corn producers. Since 1995, they have received subsidies that approach close to $76 billion dollars (http:// farm. ewg.org/progdetail.php?fips=00000&progcode=corn).

As a result, the yearly corn production continues to increase and corn is sold on the market at a cost below the true cost of production.

Because of how cheap this commodity has become, corn (which is high in omega 6) now forms the main component of most animal feed, replacing grasses (high in omega 3) and grains that had long been the traditional natural food source for cattle.

Taking advantage of the abundance and its cheap price, scientist began to break down the corn into its basic molecular components, using them in the manufacture of a variety of substances. This has resulted in the fact that over 90% of all the products we buy today contain some element of corn.

While we all know corn is increasingly used as fuel for vehicles, you may be surprised to know that components of corn is used in creating everything from make-up to batteries.

On October 28th, 2010, National Geographic News reported that chemical analysis of products obtained from fast food franchise establishments revealed that in some form, corn made up a main ingredient of most of the products sold—meat, especially.

While corn is used in animal feed and as an inexpensive meat and food filler, one of the biggest uses for corn has been in the creation of high fructose corn syrup (HFCS).

High Fructose Corn Syrup

Since the 1970's, HFCS has been used in increasing amounts as both a sweetener and preservative. It is found in a majority of the products we consume today. An article in the April 2004 issue of the American Journal of Clinical Nutrition stated that between 1970 and 1990, the consumption of HFCS increased over 1,000%.

The reason for the increase in the use of corn based HFCS has to do with the increased cost associated with table sugar. Sugar cane production quotas, import tariffs on foreign sugar and the subsidies of U.S. corn have all contributed to increasing the price of cane sugar. Consequently, HFCS became a less costly sweetener and sugar alternative.

High fructose corn syrup is any corn syrup that has undergone some enzymatic process to convert its glucose content into fructose. This produces products of varying degrees of sweetness. Currently in the United States, the most commonly available varieties of high fructose corn syrup are HFCS 55 (55% fructose and 42% glucose) and HFCS 42 (42% fructose and 53% glucose).

HFCS is a cheap sweetener found in most processed foods. It is a high calorie substance that gives sweetness to soft drinks, cereals, cookies, baked goods and many other products we consume.

On average, 10% of the total calories we consume derive from high fructose corn syrup. This is an important factor to consider in the health related epidemics such as obesity and diabetes that is present in the United States and other countries. Compared to other countries, however, we consume more HFCS on a per capita basis.

In addition to the increasing quantities of HFCS consumed, some believe that HFCS contributes to obesity because the fructose in the HCFS does not cause the normal insulin response that occurs after consuming regular table sugar. As a result, there is no suppression of our appetite, allowing us to keep eating and consuming more calories (L. Ferder, M.D. Ferder, & F. Inserra (2010). "The role of high-fructose corn syrup in metabolic syndrome and hypertension". Current Hypertension Report 12: 105-112).

Fructose metabolism also skips the normal carbohydrate metabolism pathways. As a result, <u>fructose metabolism functions and acts as a starting material for the synthesis of fatty acid, which increases fat deposition over time.</u>

Conditions associated with chronic HFCS consumption include non-alcoholic fatty liver disease (NAFL), which the most common cause of chronic liver disease in the United States affecting as much as 30% of the population. One of the main causes of NAFL is an excessive consumption of carbohydrates and/or fats, which results in producing elevated levels of blood glucose, insulin secretion and triglyceride levels.

While the increase in cases of NAFL is due to both the fructose and glucose components of HFCS, findings of studies carried out in humans, have recommended that fructose be avoided in the prevention and treatment of NAFLD (M. Allocca & C. Selmi (2010). "Emerging nutritional treatments for nonalcoholic fatty liver disease". Nutrition, diet therapy, and the liver: 131-146).

In addition to non-alcoholic fatty liver disease, HFCS is considered to be a cause of and be associated with many other chronic conditions and illnesses.

A more recent and important concern with HFCS has to due with the finding of trace amounts of mercury in samples of products made with HFCS. The mercury found is believed to have resulted from sodium hydroxide and hydrochloric acid—two chemicals used during the manufacturing and production of HFCS (Mercury from chlor-alkali plants: measured concentrations in food product sugar, Renee Dufaul (http://www.ehjournal.net/content/8/1/2).

Over the last several years, HFCS has received so much negative press that many individuals are choosing to simply decrease HFCS consumption and are avoiding food items that contain it. As a result, products that have traditionally been manufactured with high fructose corn syrup have switched away from it and stopped using it. Sugar made from cane and beets is making a come back as the natural sweetener of choice. Manufacturers are taking advantage of the consumer demand by even re-labeling their products as "HFCS free".

Popular diets for weight reduction

One only has to look at the many diets contained in magazines and the tabloid papers at the check out aisles of your local grocery store or food market to recognize that we are saturated and bombarded with thousands of fad diets. Many of them proclaim to be "revolutionary" in helping you achieve weight loss.

If you go to the nearest bookstore or online bookseller, you will find multiple sections with hundreds of books on diets and the latest treatments in weight loss. Not only diet books, diet pills, weight-reducing powders, and liquid concoctions are available as well. Some even brag and make the claim to produce weight loss without exercise.

While many diets do work, many simply miss the mark. Others just lighten your wallet instead of your weight.

We are over saturated and bombarded with popular diets because they generate billions of dollars a year in revenue, catering to a generation interested in quick and effortless results.

This diet industry has been progressively growing in size and in revenues since the 1970's. According to Marketdata, sales of diet or weight loss products in 2007, was nearly $55 billion. It was forecasted to top $80 billion in 2010. Other quoted diet and weight loss product sales numbers ranged from $40 to $90 billion a year, and increasing with each consecutive year. We spend a fortune on diets but we get mixed results. Studies have shown that the majority of those who successfully loose weight while on diets usually regain the weight in a short amount of time.

The best diet is the one the works for you long term.

There is no one diet that will provide the same weight loss results for everyone who tries it.

But have you ever asked yourselves why there are so many different diets and so many variations of diets?

The bottom line is that every type of diet in existence produces the same end result—weight loss—by means of reducing the amount of calories you consume. Period!

You too can create your own diet, by choosing to consume less calories. Eat smaller portions of foods that are more filling and with time you will see yourself getting thinner.

The main differences between the different diets, typically depends on which component of the macronutrient is being decreased or eliminated. (We will soon learn about macronutrients).

All diets are similar in that they reduce calories as well as the portion size to be consumed. And more importantly, they ALL require exercise.

Traditionally, fad diets have been popular diets based on the reduction or total elimination of the fat component. The Ornish™ and Pritikin™ diets can be found in this category.

Not too long ago, fat was the macronutrient being blamed for most of society's health problems. In fact, there was a time in America when all types of dietary fat developed such a bad reputation that it was even considered as public health enemy number one. Taking advantage of this belief, food companies began to develop, produce and sell new lines of fat free or low fat food products. Soon, the grocery aisles were full of these newly created "reduced fat" or "fat-free" products, which many people incorrectly believed to be a healthy alternative food choice. Due to clever nationwide marketing and advertising campaigns, the demand for these new products shot up dramatically.

For the first time, many people were consuming these products guilt free, because they believed that no fat meant that they wouldn't become fat. Eventually people did get fat, and increased in weight and size, only now at an even faster rate than before.

What had happened was that by reducing or eliminating the fat component (concept similar to all elimination diets), the flavoring, texture and consistency of the food had to be replaced with added carbohydrates in the form of sugars and refined flour. Besides being high in calories, these foods were of low nutritional quality and messes up our insulin secretion and metabolism. Because people were eating more cookies, cakes and various other fat free foods and gaining even more weight, some doctors began to think that perhaps the problem was not the fat component. Perhaps it was the carbohydrate content that was responsible for weight gain.

Others went further and began to associate and recognize the composition of these highly refined, and processed food items to be the principal factor directly responsible for the development of chronic inflammation, which leads to obesity.

As a result there was a change of mind and change of heart, with the realization that a good weight loss diet had nothing to do with fats.

Instead, the new belief was that fat consumption was actually not bad, but beneficial for weight reduction. Diets that where high in protein and fat and low in carbohydrates soon followed, and became the rage for many years to come. Protein only diets, in the form of liquid protein diets, became popular in the 1970's but quickly fell out of favor, after many people died of complications associated with renal failure and kidney damage. This was a direct consequence of the type of protein used in this fad diet.

High fat diets, on the other hand, have been around for over 20 years and continue to exist today. The Adkins Diet™ is a perfect example.

With some tweaking, the South Beach Diet™ was born and became another very popular diet. On the South Beach Diet™, after an initial phase of elimination of certain types of foods, the diet slowly introduces and includes good choices of all three macronutrient classes of foods. This allows the dieter more choice in their meal selections.

Eating protein causes a feeling of fullness so you tend to eat less, reducing the amount of calories consumed. Protein and fat also produces a state of ketosis that acts as a diuretic. This increases the elimination of fluid in the body, resulting in weight loss at least in the short term.

Again, all these types of popular diets calculate and control the caloric content of the food item and more importantly, the portion size.

Other popular diets include the raw foods diet, macrobiotic diet, and blood type diet. Followers of these diets believe the particular foods consumed, interact better with their bodies, producing less toxicity and improving digestion. I can't disagree.

Some diets have celebrity spokespeople who endorse the products and actually achieve dramatic results.

My concern with some of these pre-packaged meals is the high preservative and chemical content they contain. While they reduce portion size and calories, the majority of these meals are manufactured weeks before and preserved with potential obesogene causing chemicals and substances whose long term consequences are as of yet unknown. This allows them to be kept on shelves for varying periods of time. <u>In my opinion, the only thing that pre-packaged boxed weight loss diet systems provide is convenience.</u>

The human chorionic gonadotropin (hCG) diet is currently a popular fad diet. This "diet" consists of a medically supervised administration of a hormone (hCG) that is produced during pregnancy by the developing embryo and later by the placenta. The principal component of this diet however is, an ultra-low calorie diet. A 500 calorie-a-day diet. What I find amazing is that intelligent people actually buy into this scam, and pay hundreds to thousands of dollars for it. Men and women not only allowing themselves to be given a pregnancy hormone, but not recognizing that it's the associated low calorie diet that is responsible for the weight loss. In addition, the FDA has called this diet a fraud and ineffective and both the AMA and Journal of Clinical Nutrition have proclaimed it to neither safe nor an effective weight loss practice.

In addition to the diets mentioned above, there are literally thousands of other diets around.

Some work better for certain individuals, while others produce no results.

Whatever diet you choose to try, you need to be careful and do your homework first.

Remember also that frequently after ending these diets, the mind-body connection goes into overdrive, causing even greater food urges. This causes one to indulge and overeat, even when not truly hungry. What eventually results is a "yo-yo" effect, where one tends to lose and regain weight cyclically, on a regular basis, seemingly gaining more weight with each cycle.

I equate the different types of available diets to the various gasoline formulations available. These range from regular to high octane to diesel for different engine types.

A fuel that works well for one, will not necessarily work for another, and may even be damaging because individual needs and characteristics differs from person to person.

Likewise, I believe that as individuals, we either have a genetic predisposition, or we acquire some type of resistance throughout life, perhaps as a result of exposure to a substance or toxin, that makes the components of a particular diet produce results for one person and not the other. Similar perhaps to the role of insulin or leptin resistance, that was previously mentioned. An interesting diet concept that will be left for the field of genomics to unravel and figure out.

This is why I believe there is no one, ideal, universal diet that works for all. There are too many variables that make up our own uniqueness and individuality to simply buy into any of the weight loss hype claimed and sold on infomercials.

"One size does not fit all."

Instead, I echo what my wife and other registered dieticians have been recommending, which is a diet where you eat from all macronutrient categories without exclusion as long as the food choices are healthy, and natural.

What is certain is that there has always been and will continue to be confusion among people in regards to the kind of diet that is most effective in reducing weight and maintaining it off.

This confusion is made only more difficult because the majority of western—trained, allopathic physicians (such as myself), never received any formal nutritional education and may be of little or no help to their patients.

It is sad, but nutrition and diet, so basic and fundamental a subject that is associated with wellness and disease and is as important as anatomy, chemistry and physiology, is not formally required in our medical schools or taught in residency training.

In conclusion, most of the popular diets are based on calorie reduction.

They require exercise.

Many are typically consumed or maintained for a short time, limited by their cost, boredom, lack of variety or achievement of the short-term weight loss goal.

A better choice would be to eat a wide selection of more natural, fresh, less processed foods.

Food as Medicine

The definition of a drug is: <u>"any substance that when absorbed into the body of a living organism, alters normal bodily function"</u>. Doesn't food do that?

Per the many examples mentioned previously throughout this book, we know without any doubt that the type, quality and quantity of food we eat affects our health and wellbeing.

The eminent medical historian Henry E. Sigerist once noted, "There is no sharp borderline between food and drug," and that both dietetic and pharmacological therapies were "born of instinct" (Sigerist, H., 1951. A History of Medicine, Vol. I, Primitive and Archaic Medicine. Oxford University Press, New York. Sigerist, H).

The concept of utilizing food as a medicine is not a new one.

For over 5000 years, medical practitioners of whole body medical systems (such as the Indian medical practice of Ayurveda and traditional Chinese medicine) have used food as a medicine. The ancient Greeks and Romans wrote extensively about the subject. It was Hippocrates, considered the father of medicine, who wrote: "Let your food be your medicine, and your medicine be your food."

Ayurvedic medicine believes that the right combination, proportions and quality of the food we eat, is the first step in achieving a balanced and healthy life.

According to Ayurveda teachings, the food we eat on a regular basis becomes a medicine when properly individualized and optimized to meet the constitutional needs and particular imbalances that need to be corrected. If food is improperly used or abused, over time it can become a cause of many diseases. Ayurvedic pharmacology utilizes herbs, minerals, oils, spices, and other naturally occurring substances, as well as animal products, either alone or in combination, as a basis of their healing.

This medical teaching, that continues to be practiced in many parts of the world today, is as relevant and perhaps even more important today then it has ever has been.

Traditional Chinese Medicine (TCM) is over 4000 years old, and had its origins from the Chinese Taoist philosophy. According to this philosophy, man is an essential and integral part of nature's energy. To be distanced or separated from it results in physical, mental or emotional disharmony. Thus, TCM views disease as an expression of the individual being out of balance with the fundamental laws of nature.

Any time an individual is out of balance, development of illness is favored. The concept of polar opposites, referred to as Yin and Yang, present in all objects, is an important concept of TCM.

Healing, therefore, consists of different modalities that include movement, meditation, dietary and lifestyle counseling, acupuncture and/or herbs.

They are all used with the purpose of trying to restore balance and harmony to a dysfunctional body, mind, or spirit.

The Yellow Emperor's Classic of Internal Medicine, written around 3000 BC, was the most important medical text in forming the basis of Chinese food therapy. Food, as per this ancient medical textbook, was also noted to play a dominant role in a person's health and wellbeing.

Traditional Chinese Medicine classifies food into four main food groups and an additional five group classification according to the taste, unique nature, and characteristics of the particular food. The Yellow Emperor's Classic text, also described the importance of consuming the right amounts or proportions of both Ying and Yang foods, in order to keep the body in balance and free of disease.

In addition to the importance and central role food had as part of each individuals treatment plan, practitioners of these traditional medical systems also recognized that each patient as a unique individual. Each individual therefore required their own personalized treatment plan that takes into account the uniqueness of their mind, body, physical and spiritual make up. Factors, which need to be addressed in order to be able to restore balance, harmony and health.

These traditional medical systems share with Integrative Medicine, the belief that <u>the body has an innate ability to heal itself.</u> Sadly, this is a belief that is not taught or even mentioned in conventional Western medical curriculums.

With a rich and extensive history that allows us to trace and document the overwhelming use of food and nutrition to preserve health as well as treat illness and disease, it is rather sad and surprising that, as a society have come to rely on expensive chemicals, and drugs for all that ails us. We give food little or no consideration in the healing process, let alone utilize it as a medication.

PART TWO

Elimination Diet

As we just mentioned, food can be used to heal people, and at other times it can cause illness. There are many illnesses and medical conditions in which withholding food or excluding a particular macronutrient component is not only recommended, it is necessary to achieve optimum health. Diets that eliminate a certain food macronutrient component to obtain a health benefit are referred to as "elimination diets".

You've already learned that weight-reducing diets available are a form of an elimination diet. This is because a certain component (whether it be fat, protein, carbohydrate or combination of these) is completely eliminated from the particular diet. This type of an elimination diet however, is done to achieve weight loss, and not prescribed as a direct medical treatment for a particular illness. This is the main difference between a weight loss diet and an elimination diet employed for the treatment of a particular medical condition.

The following are a few examples of medical conditions that employ elimination diets as part of their medical treatment.

Gluten sensitivity/Celiac disease.

An NIH study from 2004 found that 1 out of 133 Americans have gluten sensitivity (intolerance), which equals to ½ to 1% of the U.S. population.

The great majority of these individuals, which some have estimated to be as high as 90%, remain undiagnosed because they present with or manifest atypical symptoms. As you already know, many of these individuals may be considered gluten sensitive because they have symptoms suggestive of the disease but negative or "normal" gluten screening tests.

Celiac disease is an autoimmune disorder, in which our body's immune system turns on itself and is "activated" against the protein component found in wheat, barley and rye. Eventually, Celiac disease can produce damage to the lining of the small intestine, which leads to problems of absorption of nutrients and the development of digestive symptoms.

Sufferers of Celiac disease and gluten intolerance can develop deficiencies of iron, calcium, and fat-soluble vitamins. As a result, patients frequently develop iron deficiency anemia, osteopenia and osteoporosis. Irritability, failure to thrive, bloating, constipation, abdominal pain, fatigue, headaches, and even rashes which are all non-specific symptoms that can be experienced by gluten sensitive patients.

Because of this, gluten sensitivity or intolerance can frequently be misdiagnosed as other illnesses, resulting in extensive work-ups.

Physicians and patients need to consider the possibility of food as a possible culprit with any non-specific systemic ailment especially ones that affect the gastro-intestinal tract, as the symptoms of Celiac disease and gluten sensitivity evolve with time.

Treatment for this condition does not relay on medications but rather on eliminating wheat, barley and rye, as well as products that contain wheat based substances from the diet, for life.

Inflammatory bowel disease (IBD) is a group of inflammatory conditions that affect the small intestine and colon. Two separate entities make up IBD and they are ulcerative colitis (UC) and Crohn's disease (CD).

Patients with UC have been found to have significantly higher concentrations of hydrogen sulphide in their intestine. The major dietary sources of sulphur are those found in high protein foods such as red meats, dairy products, nuts and preservatives found in processed foods.

Crohn's disease, the other entity that makes up IBD, is associated with diets high that are high in carbohydrates and refined sugars. Consumption of these substances precedes the development of the condition in the majority of cases. Modified fats like trans-fats may be a contributing cause of this condition (Journal of clinical gastroenterology 19(2):166-71 Dietary and other risk factors of ulcerative colitis. A case-control study in Japan).

In addition to medications, treatment of both of these conditions is comprised of an elimination diet, which removes the particular causative food component (protein in UC and carbohydrates and sugars in Crohns) from the diet.

A reduction or elimination of protein is also part of the treatment of individuals with renal failure.

Childhood asthma is frequently related to, and made worse by, the ingestion of dairy products. In addition to medications, avoidance of and/or substitution of cow milk has resulted in resolution of many asthma symptoms.

Even the elimination or reduction of micronutrients forms an important component of a person's medical treatment. This is the case with salt restriction or elimination in those with congestive heart failure and/or a weak heart muscle. Salt restriction also forms the dietary treatment for the control of elevated blood pressure.

Patients with irritable bowel syndrome (IBS), (not to be confused with the previously mentioned, inflammatory bowel disease (IBD), also report development of symptoms in association with the ingestion of certain types of food items. By removing these foods from their diet, they can remain and live symptom-free.

The primary medical treatment of IBS will include avoidance and elimination of potential food triggers, which include flour, dairy products, sugar and other fermented, poorly absorbed carbohydrates.

In a condition called eosinophilic esophagitis (a condition that is associated with gastro-esophageal reflux or heartburn), an elimination diet that removes food allergens, has been found to be the preferred treatment in its resolution.

These are just a few of the many illness and medical conditions that are benefited by a change in the food consumed.

Oligoantigenic diets

Oligo, in Greek, simply means "a few" and antigen is a substance that causes an immune response. An oligoantigenic diet is one in which foods that are potentially associated with allergies or different food intolerances are removed from the diet. It's not so much a macronutrient being removed, as it is particular allergen substance contained in the food, such as toxin, dye, chemical additive or nutrient component contained in the particular food item. What results is a sort of trial and error elimination of any one of several potential substances believed to be the cause of an acute inflammatory reaction and/or illness caused by its ingestion.

Common allergen producing substances include dairy items, eggs, corn, soy, wheat, peanut, shellfish, chocolates or citrus products. After the food items are eliminated from the diet, they are slowly re-introduced one by one in order to narrow the culprit food item causing the adverse effect. This forms the basis of an oligoantigenic diet.

As previously mentioned, most pediatricians know that very common triggers for and cause of childhood asthma are cows milk and dairy products. Often times, asthma is a frequent manifestation of lactose intolerance. <u>Mammals are typically the only species that drink milk after birth and while very young.</u> (It is interesting to note that as a result, the gene that is responsible for our ability to digest and process lactose slowly deactivates after infancy and as we grow older, resulting in lactose intolerance in later life).

Many asthmatic children dramatically improve their symptoms and even remain asthma free by simply removing dairy products from their diets—often times even without having a positive allergy panel reaction, as these diagnostic tests are rarely exact. (As you already know by now, a "normal", negative or non-reactive allergy test should never be considered definitive, or conclusive. This is especially true in the presence of persistent symptoms that occurs in individuals in response to certain food items).

The use of oligoantigenic diets have been investigated in many medical conditions including migraines, epilepsy, and hyperactivity states. They have been successfully used in the reduction of complex and problematic symptoms in many of these conditions.

In a study published in the medical journal Lancet, 76 overactive children were treated with an oligoantigenic diet. Sixty-two of them, (81%) achieved improvement their hyperactivity and a normal range of behavior was achieved in 21 of the children. Other symptoms such as headaches, abdominal pain, and fits, also improved.

Twenty-eight of the children who improved then completed a double-blind, crossover, placebo-controlled trial in which foods thought to provoke symptoms were re-introduced.

In conclusion, this study revealed that 48 foods were suspected of causing the states of hyperactivity, including most noticeably, artificial colorants (Controlled trial of oligoantigenic treatment in the hyperkinetic syndrome. (The Lancet, Volume 325, Issue 8428, Pages 540-545)).

In another oligoantigenic trial, 78 children with hyperactivity were placed on an oligoantigenic elimination diet. Fifty-nine improved in behavior during the open phase of the trial. The results of the crossover trial showed that provoking foods (those believed to cause symptoms), significantly worsened ratings of behavior, as well as caused impaired psychological test performance. It may be that a certain proportion of the increasing cases of hyperactivity and attention deficit disorders being recognized, share a dietary component that may include food allergies as triggers or sustainer of symptoms.

Over the last 20-30 years, migraine headaches have increased between 6 and 11% in children and from 25% to 40% in adults. Again, dietary factors, such as increased coffee intake, aspartame or other chemicals in diet drinks, food additives, and underage drinking are possible explanations (Mar 25, 2003 Millichap JG, Yee MM. The diet factor in pediatric and adolescent migraine. Pediatr Neurol 2003;28:9-15).

Another study evaluated the role of oligoantigenic diets in 63 children with epilepsy. Forty-five of these children with epilepsy had associated migraine or hyperkinetic behavior. Of the 45 children who had epilepsy with the associated symptoms, 25 ceased to have seizures and 11 had fewer seizures during oligoantigenic diet therapy (Oligoantigenic diet treatment of children with epilepsy and migraine. Egger J, Carter CM, Soothill JF, Wilson J. J Pediatr. 1989 Jan;114(1):51-8).

Other oligoantigenic studies have shown that cow milk and cheeses made from cow milk caused headaches in most of the patients in one study, but none complained of headaches after substituting the cheese with products made with goat milk. This is another example of our body's immune system being triggered by a certain substance. In this case, it was most likely a protein in cow milk. Similar immune responses occur in response to other irritants or allergens, which then continue to produce non-specific symptoms throughout life and even result in many chronic conditions.

High-fat, ketogenic diet

In mentioning another example that illustrates the importance of our nutrition and the foods we consume, with relation to the functions of the body, I will discuss a highly specialized, rarely mentioned, medically prescribed diet, called a high fat, ketogenic diet. This type of diet has been around since the 1920's. It is a diet used in some cases of intractable seizures, and one that should not be consumed or tried by the general public.

It was developed after a reduction in the number of epileptic seizures was noted, with periods of fasting. With time, fasting was replaced by the consumption of saturated fats, as it was found that the breakdown of fats produces similar chemical changes in the brain.

This diet is utilized as a treatment option for children with refractory epilepsy that has been unable to be controlled with medications.

It consists of replacing a healthy balanced diet to one that consists of 80% or greater of saturated fats.

This is a diet that goes against everything we have been taught and what we, as physicians and health care providers, have been recommending to our patients. Pediatric neurologists, however, have found success in decreasing the numbers and duration of epileptic seizures in patients with refractory epilepsy utilizing this type of diet.

It works as follows:

The cells in our bodies, especially our brain cells (neurons), need glucose for their normal functions. By consuming a diet high in fats, the normal glucose based fuel source is switched and in its place, the needed energy source for normal functions is derived from fats. The breakdown of the fats produces substances called ketones and produces a state of ketosis. This is a condition similar to what can occur in uncontrolled diabetics who are insulin dependant when there is insufficient insulin to appropriately metabolize and breakdown high levels of glucose.

In ketosis, fat is used, broken down and metabolized to provide the needed energy required for bodily functions, resulting in increased fat metabolism. Ketones, in turn produces a range of different metabolic changes, including reducing blood pH. Although it is not yet known exactly how this state of ketosis causes a reduction in seizure episodes, children placed on high fat diets have demonstrated significant improvement in terms of reduced seizure rates, frequencies and duration.

Another example of the impact food and nutrition has on our bodily functions.

These are just a few examples of the different conditions that have shown impressive and significant responses to a dietary change. Unfortunately, many people, including physicians, frequently fail to recognize the possible relationships between common illnesses and our food and nutritional choices. In large part this has occurred because of a lack of understanding of basic nutrition, as well as our dependence on medications to cure all that ails us.

Makes you wonder why government doesn't do more to fund research into the dietary treatment of disease.

The anti-inflammatory diet

The diet and the nutrition we choose is vital in preserving, maintaining and recovering our health and wellness, and should be considered a key component and be included as part of any medical treatment.

According to the American College of Medicine:

"There is increasing scientific evidence of positive health effects from diets that are high in fruits, vegetables, legumes, and whole grains, and that include fish, nuts, and low-fat dairy products. Such diets need not be restricted in total fat as long as they preclude an excess of calories and emphasize predominantly vegetable oils that are low in saturated fats and free of partially hydrogenated oils. The traditional Mediterranean diet, in which olive oil is the principal source of fat, encompasses these dietary characteristics".

An anti-inflammatory type diet takes its foundation and principal from a traditional Mediterranean diet, as well from the diets of the Inuits Indians in Greenland. Both diets are high in good fats and composed of natural, healthy food choices.

<u>What is to be avoided with anti-inflammatory type diets are refined and processed foods that are loaded with chemicals and preservatives.</u>

The anti-inflammatory diet consists of avoidance of saturated fats, sugars and foods that are of high calorie and poor nutritional value.

<u>An anti-inflammatory diet is one diet that allows us to use food to our advantage</u>, by keeping us healthy and helps in decreasing our risk of developing chronic illnesses.

This is the way we were meant to eat and should eat, from the cradle to the grave.

An anti-inflammatory type diet should form the basic nutrition of individuals who are interested in staying healthy and maintaining wellness. It consists of food that nourishes our bodies and our soul, instead of fattening our bellies and butts.

Anti-inflammatory foods are packed with vitamins, minerals and natural chemical substances called phytonutrients that are natures' very own antioxidants.

Anti-inflammatory foods are those that are whole, fresh, unprocessed, and grown as organic as possible without pesticides or other chemical additives. They are foods that are typically grown and produced in smaller quantities, for naturally longer periods of time and under natural conditions. Foods that are the exact opposite of the processed, highly refined, mass-produced foodstuffs we have been consuming over the last several decades.

Anti-inflammatory diets go back to basic nutrition 101, and requires common sense.

"No illness that can be treated by diet

should be treated by any other means"

~ Moses Maimonides (1135-1204)

Seven Countries Study

Ancel Keys, PhD. Is the name of one those rare scientist and medical researchers that no one has ever heard of, but whose contributions to our understanding of health and nutrition, truly makes him a giant among many.

Dr. Keys was the first to associate and make a connection between the ingestion of certain types of fats and cholesterol with the development of cardiovascular diseases. He recognized this association after studying the high rates of cardiovascular diseases amongst American businessmen in the mid 1940's who, at the time, were considered to be among the best fed and best nourished people when compared to those in post-war Europe. Interestingly enough, people in post-war Europe had lower cardiovascular disease rates due to the reduced food supplies.

Dr. Keys first started to write about the benefits of a low fat, healthy food choice diet (similar to a Mediterranean type diet) at that time. It wasn't until the 1990's, with the increased rates of heart disease in industrialized nations, that people started to take notice of his vast work.

To further test his observation of increased fat consumption leading to increased cardiovascular disease, a large prospective study called the "Seven Country Study" was started in 1958. This was the first study to examine the relationships between lifestyle, diet, coronary heart disease and stroke in different populations from various regions of the world.

It not only identified causes of coronary heart disease and stroke, but more importantly it was the first study to demonstrate that an individual's risk could be modified with dietary and lifestyle changes.

It was the Seven Country Study that demonstrated that increased cholesterol consumption increases cardiovascular risk. It also showed an association between increased cholesterol levels as well as being overweight or obese, with increased mortality from cancer. All these associations are still being demonstrated today. The findings of this study also gave us what is known as the Mediterranean diet.

Mediterranean diet.

So what exactly is the Mediterranean diet, why the hoopla and does it really work?

The Mediterranean diet is named after the countries around the Mediterranean Sea, where most of the beneficial effects of lifestyle and food patterns where first noticed by Dr. Keys, while he was stationed in Southern Italy. The diet is based on the typical food patterns of Southern Italy, Greece, Crete and Spain observed during the 1960's. Sadly, many of these same regions are suffering today from rates of chronic illnesses approaching those of the West, due mainly to the adoption of a Western dietary and lifestyle habits.

The anti-inflammatory diet, just like the Mediterranean diet, is based on fresh foods such as vegetables, fruits, cereals, nuts, legumes, dairy products including cheeses and yogurts that are locally produced, as well as wines, lean red meats in reduced amounts, naturally raised chicken in minimal to moderate amounts, fresh fish and fats (mainly from olive oil). All these foods are as fresh, unprocessed, unrefined and as close to their natural state as possible in order for us to benefit from their high nutrient content. Foods that today are considered organically grown, and as natural as possible.

So the hoopla associated with the Mediterranean diet has to due to the fact that it was one of the first "diets" that changed and reversed chronic illnesses, which developed as a result of poor food consumption.

At the time the Mediterranean diet was first described, the US was in the middle of a growing economy and expansion. It was a post-war, post-hardship, and post sacrifice era. Seemingly overnight, our country went from rationing and scarcity to abundance, drive-ins and carhops. Because of this prosperity and the consequential changes with time of our food production, quality and eating habits, we became a society that pretty much revolved around eating. Food was no longer used to nourish us properly. It was now abundant, cheap and readily available. These changes, added to an increasingly sedentary lifestyle, incrementally gave way to the tremendous rise in obesity, illness and disease.

But what was old is new again.

A re-emergence and interest in healthier diets and nutrition is making a comeback. As a result, a resurgence and renewed interest in the Mediterranean diet and other anti-inflammatory diets are gaining popularity once again.

These types of diets are relevant today because, as explained, there is a direct association and correlation between our diet and chronic inflammation and illnesses.

Quick fixes

As a practicing physician in the United States during the 21st century, more of us have become specialists in diseases. Notice that we are no longer trained to be healers, as were Hippocrates, Galen, Hopkins and the other great practioners of our profession that preceded us. We have become, "one size fits all", disease specialists, becoming even increasingly super-specialized and focusing on the treatment of one body system.

As a cardiologist, I know a lot about the heart and cardiovascular disease. I have specialized training in nuclear cardiology, able to interpret cardiac function at an atomic level. There are now cardiologists that specialize in lipids and cholesterol. Others that specialize in the treatment of weak heart muscles or (cardiomyopathies) and still others that only do angioplasties, stents and intra-coronary procedures. Ask us to explain to you details about your headache or migraine and well, for that I would need to send you to a neurologist. Upset stomach or digestive issues? I really don't have too much time to spend on something I wasn't trained in, so let me refer you to a gastroenterologist. Sore joints? Call the rheumatologist. And so on. The practice of medicine has become fractionated. We are specializing in parts, instead of treating the whole.

Not only is it easier to refer patients out to other specialists, many physicians refer to other specialists to cover themselves from potential malpractice lawsuits.

It seems that as patients, we go from one type of doctor to another type of doctor until we finally find out what is wrong, or we get tired and give up, or our health insurance denies any additional benefits. I often feel sad and embarrassed that our healthcare system treats patients as though they were parts on a conveyer belt, going around in circles form one provider to the next only to end up at the same place they started, with no resolution or improvement of their ailment.

Does any of this seem too familiar to you?

America's healthcare is the best money can buy, if you have a boatload of cash. It is also the best in the world at treating life threatening traumatic injuries, and any delicate, complex pathology that requires specialized instrumentation and training. What we are deficient at and lack is in the more common, everyday management of reversible ailments that lead to chronic illnesses. Conditions, that makes up the bulk of our medical practices.

Consequently, we physicians have lost touch with the art of healing. This is sad because I am reminded that healing begins within our patients' mind, and involves their heart and soul. We don't treat the patient as a whole human being, instead, we outsource to others.

As physicians and healthcare providers, we are also under pressure to prescribe the latest, greatest "life-altering" drug that comes to market, continuing the cycle of pill pushing over something as benign as lifestyle change.

People in the United States also seem to be addicted to medications, or at least they have accepted drugs as a cure-all. Not only do we treat everything with pills, many patients honestly believe that health and wellness can be found at the bottom of a bottle.

It's time to stop this madness.

What if we could all start to take control of our own health and healthcare, without having to rely on doctors, nurses, healthcare providers or others?

What if we had the knowledge and tools available to make simple changes that would lead us to better health and wellness? What if the changes could decrease and limit the need for doctor visits and prescription drugs? Wouldn't that be worthwhile? Shouldn't we all be able to live this kind of life?

If you think we should, that is why learning about the importance of nutrition is so valuable for the entire family.

Following a diet that is based on fresh, natural, and unprocessed foods, typical of an anti-inflammatory, or Mediterranean type diet is the key to start our path to wellness.

It is the one thing WE can decide to do for ourselves. Changing our eating habits also empowers us to be an active participant in our own health and wellbeing. There is no greater gift than that.

Our nutrition and the quality of our foods are more relevant and important now than they have ever been. Unlike many other treatments, healthy diets are affordable and have no side effects. Best of all, we can be as intense or as flexible as we want.

As a result of our understanding of healthy, natural diets, we have come to recognize that not all macronutrients or food items are bad. These diets have shown us is the importance of incorporating all macronutrients—fats, carbohydrates, and proteins—in our diets.

These diets show us that we don't need to avoid anything, as health is maintained by consuming foods and nutrients from all three, food categories. What is important, however, is to learn to differentiate between good fats and bad fats, good carbs and bad carbs, and good proteins and bad proteins. Again, it is about choosing and allowing foods to work for us. These foods provide their nutrients, satisfy our hunger and decrease inflammation due to their contents of natural anti-oxidants and health promoting phytonutrients.

Remember that at one time, fat was considered public enemy number one. It was avoided at all costs, which led to the reduced fat and fat free craze. As we all know now, that didn't turn out so well.

We need to switch from the bad fats, such as saturated and man-made trans fats, (all too prevalent in the commercial food industry), to good fats, such as olive oil, flax seed oil and other omega 3 oils.

We don't need to avoid or eliminate carbohydrates; we just need to learn and know the difference between those that break down quickly (such as white breads, white rice, pastries, and sugary meals) and those that break down slowly and more consistently (like we get with whole grain or wheat bread, black rice and brown rice).

Lastly, we can choose lean red meats, white meats, fish, or plant sources for our protein instead of the large amount of steak, burgers and other saturated fat containing red meat sources we consume.

We also need to remember that most processed fast foods contain chemicals, additives, pesticides and other substances that have been shown to cause allergies and obesity. This is also true for the many pre-packaged, mass-produced "diet" foods some celebrities endorse.

Many of us can find it very confusing and overwhelming to understand what constitutes a healthy diet. What are we to eat?

We are constantly being bombarded on a daily basis with mixed weight loss messages.

This is because of the many weight loss products and diets that falsely guarantee fast and easy weight loss, some, even without the need for exercise.

The bottom line is to avoid extremes and recognize that what our bodies need is consistently healthy nutrition in order to maintain proper health.

There are no magic bullets or magic remedies.

There will always be trade-offs with most weight loss gimmicks. We may quickly loose weight today, only to suffer untoward effects years from now, as a result of the foods and diets loaded with chemicals we eat today.

Remember that weight loss ultimately affects every organ system in the body. Remember also that food nourishes all the cells of the body. The eventual yo-yo <u>effects from rapid weight loss and weight gain is in itself another inflammatory stimulant</u> that leads to even greater eventual weight gain.

Although most studies done on the long term effects of the various popular weight loss and fad diets show a return of the weight that was previously lost after terminating such a diet, a Mediterranean or anti-inflammatory diet utilizing natural, whole foods, allows you to maintain the weight off. Most importantly, an anti-inflammatory type diet has been proven to reverse heart disease and many other chronic illnesses.

Imagine eating your way to a healthier life. What a concept!

I'll briefly mention that the term "French Paradox" has been used to describe the Mediterranean diet by some people. This is based on the fact that it is a diet in which a large quantity of fats are consumed; yet results in rates of cardiovascular diseases that are low when compared to the typical Western diets, where similar quantities of fats are also consumed.

In my opinion, this association of the Mediterranean diet with the French Paradox is incorrect. This is because while the Mediterranean diet consists of good quality, unsaturated fats, the typical French diet, consists of mainly saturated fats. Both however, result in lower incidences of cardiovascular diseases.

Again, the consumption of a diet high in saturated fat and findings of low cardiovascular and coronary artery disease is a paradox that goes against the findings of the Seven Country Study as well as the Framingham Study and the Nurses Health Study.

All 3 of which have demonstrated the associations of cardiovascular disease with risk factors that include dietary fat.

The fats consumed in a Mediterranean or anti-inflammatory diet comes mainly from olive oil, fish and plants. These fats are monounsaturated fats that are cardio-protective, as well as high in omega 3 or good fat. Reason for which there really is no paradox. We already know that not all fats are created equal.

"A doctor treats the disease, a good doctor treats the patient with disease"

~ Sir William Osler (1849-1919)

Macronutrients

As previously mentioned, all of the foods we consume can be classified into 3 main categories or classes.

These include proteins, carbohydrates and fats. Some also have included alcohol as another, fourth category of macronutrient. For our purposes, however, we will go into detail about the macronutrients that comprise items found on a typical plate of food.

These macronutrients can either be consumed as individual items like (rice—carbohydrate; soy—protein; olive oil—fat), or as we do more commonly, in a variation of combinations similar to how we eat a typical meal. Meatloaf (protein/fat) and gravy (fat), is usually served with mashed potatoes, vegetable and corn bread (all of which are carbohydrates). A pasta (carbohydrate) dinner, if served with red meat sauce (protein/fat) or Alfredo sauce (fat) and garlic bread (carbohydrate/fat). Wine, can be considered to be a form of carbohydrate.

A burger combo is typically comprised of beef (protein and fat), a soda (carbohydrate) and fries (carbohydrates fried in fat).

Next time you eat out at a restaurant, notice how items on a menu consists of a portion of protein served with sides of carbohydrates, and that most of these proteins contain fats. Fat may also be added in some form to complete the meal.

You can also try to identify the food items into their corresponding macronutrient class in order to become more familiar with what you eat. It will soon become second nature, and even reveal to you how much you fat you eat on a regular basis.

These three food categories are called macronutrients because they are the main types of foods people consume in large quantities (hence "macro").

Macronutrients are the nutrients that provide most of the calories and energy to maintain the body's metabolic functions.

1. Protein

Meats of all types, including red meats, chicken, turkey, pork, lamb, goat, duck, sausages, are all proteins derived from animal sources. Non-meat sources of proteins include soy, endaname, nuts, seeds, legumes and beans.

Proteins are organic compounds whose structure is formed by amino acids. Amino acids in turn are compounds formed by molecules of carbon, hydrogen, oxygen, nitrogen and an amine group. The organization and composition of the amino acids is driven by genetic control (that's why there are many inherited diseases, which results from a deficiency or an alteration of one or more proteins).

The digestion and breakdown of protein starts with the enzymes present in our saliva. The process begins as we chew and continues as the food bolus, as it is called, travels down to the stomach were additional gastric enzymes in the gastric juice complete the breakdown of this macronutrient into its basic component—amino acids.

Amino acids are important because they can be metabolized to produce other substances and generate energy. They can be incorporated into forming more protein molecules.

There are about 22 different types of amino acids found in food sources and in the body. Of the 22 amino acids, 14 can be synthesized, while 8 are considered and known as essential amino acids (this is because the body cannot produce them from other substances; thus they are essential and need to be acquired through the foods we eat). In addition to their important role in the formation of proteins, amino acids also play an important role in the regulation of different metabolic processes in the body. Furthermore, they can also function as enzymes.

The nutritional requirement of each of the amino acid will vary depending on the age and nutritional status of the individual.

Proteins are needed for cell growth and development of tissues and muscles, especially in growing children and pregnant women who have high metabolic rates. Among hospitalized patients and those in critical condition, especially suffering from burns, chronic illnesses and abdominal or serious digestive issues, the daily nutritional requirements for proteins are also increased. Proteins form an integral part of the cellular repair of tissues, in our body's immune function and in the synthesis of hormones. They can also be used as an energy source when carbohydrates are not available.

Proteins obtained from animal meat sources contain all the essential amino acids, while the protein foods obtained through a vegetarian diet based on plant sources, will vary in their amino acid content. This is why vegetarians need to supplement their diets with different kinds of vegetarian-based vitamins and minerals and protein supplements, especially ones that contain omega 3.

We all know that the meat from animal sources is mainly composed of protein, but we need to also recognize that any animal meat, especially red meat will also contain varying amounts of saturated fat. It is the amount of fat in the piece of meat as well as the part of the animal the meat comes from that differentiates the different cuts of meat.

It is saturated fat that contributes to elevated cholesterol levels and is a risk factor for the development of cardiovascular disease, stroke, diabetes and inflammation that gives way to various other chronic medical conditions.

Red meat should not be eliminated from the diet, but one should consider limiting its consumption to no more than once a week. Processed red meats have been associated with increased cancer rates, as are meats that are cooked until charred. The later is due to the formation of chemical substances called heterocyclic amines.

Remember also that <u>a typical "normal" serving portion consists of about 8 ounces.</u> The portion sizes we routinely get served at restaurants are servings of beef that ranges between 12-16 ounces and even larger. Many know of, or have at least heard of restaurants that typically serve up steaks or other beef portions that are well over a pound, and come accompanied by large portions side dishes. When added up, these portions tip the scales in calories and fat content. We may get quick satisfaction, but will be paying for our indulgences later in life.

A somewhat healthier alternative to red meat is white meat protein sources. These are proteins that come from turkey, pork, chicken, and fish. Chicken is the most widely consumed animal protein in the United States. We consume on average 9 billion chickens a year. Fish such as salmon, mackerel and sardines all contain less saturated fat but higher levels of the healthy omega 3 fat.

Other important sources of protein, especially for people on limited budgets or who wish to avoid meat all together, consist of legumes or beans. Beans are a rich source of protein without the saturated fat that typically accompanies red meat. Beans come in a wide variety and can be prepared in different ways so as to appeal to all tastes. Soy based products are increasing in popularity due to their high nutritional value and multiple health benefits.

Soy

Soybean has been consumed for over 5000 years in Asia. This is especially true in China, where the soybean was considered at that time, one of the 5 most sacred plants, due to its many uses, especially in its use as a nutritious food source.

Soy was introduced in Europe in the 18th century and then was brought over to the United States. It was not grown here, however, until after the First World War, during the era of the Great Depression in the 1930's as well as during the dust bowl years.

Few people remember that Henry Ford was a major investor and proponent of soy. He even fabricated a vehicle out of soy-based plastics. Today, soy continues to be well known as a plant with multiple and diverse uses. It is even used in parts that make up combines and farm equipment, which in turn are used in soy cultivation.

Soybeans and soy—derived foods are currently being consumed in increasing amounts in the United States. This is because it is a protein source that contains no saturated fat and is high in a type of omega 3 fatty acid, called alpha-linoleic acid (ALA).

Soy comes in a variety of products that most commonly includes endamame, (green soybeans cooked in their pods), ground soy made into baking flour, tofu that can be served hot and liquefied as miso soup or cold as soy milk. Many of the vegetarian type burgers, meat substitutes and other non-animal foodstuffs, may also be composed of soy.

Like corn, soy is also found as a component in many of the foods and products we use today. Soy is used in the manufacture of baby food formulas, margarine, yogurt, ice cream, and cheese.

Frequently, it is used as filler that is mixed in with beef to create burgers and other food products, as a way to reduce the cost of the meat while keeping the protein content and taste intact. Other uses for soy include adhesives, soy vodka, inks, cosmetics, lubricants, and mixed in as a component of cattle food.

The good, the mixed and the bad regarding soy.

The good.

Some have called soy a complete protein because it contains all the essential amino acids our body needs. This makes soy an important source of protein for vegans and vegetarians.

Soybeans, like colorful fruits and vegetables, contain substances called phytonutrients, which are substances found in plants that act as anti-oxidants and anti-cancer agents. The phytonutrients found in soy include many types of isoflavones, (estrogen-like chemicals), which are specific to the particular plant nutrients and is responsible for some of the plants beneficial, protective effect. Another phytonutrient found in high concentrations in soy, is phytic acid. In addition to its anti-oxidant function, phytic acid has chelation effects, resulting in a decrease in the levels of inflammation, diabetes and some cancers.

A meta-analysis published in 1995 in the New England Journal of Medicine linked the consumption of soy protein with a reduction in total cholesterol, bad cholesterol (LDL) and triglycerides levels (NEJM, vol. 333, No. 5. August 3, 1995).

Another phytonutrient in soy is sphingolipids—a natural chemical that may be helpful in reducing the risk of colon cancer (Symolon H, Schmelz E, Dillehay D, Merrill A (1 May 2004). J Nutr 134 (5): 1157-61).

The mixed

Soybeans also contain genistein and daidzein. These are two estrogen-like substances that have received mixed reviews. Some researchers and physicians believe these substances may be carcinogenic, while others seem to think they are protective against cancers. This perhaps is one of the reasons for the confusion and concerns regarding the consumption of soy, especially in post-menopausal women and those who have had breast cancer.

There have been more than 20 epidemiologic studies examining the relationship between soy intake and breast cancer risk—all with mixed results.

Two recent studies found that when soy products are consumed in childhood or in adolescence (at a time in which the breast tissue is still developing), a 25-50% reduction in breast cancer risk occurred in later adult life. This suggests a protective effect (Korde LA etal. Childhood soy intake and breast cancer risk in Asian American women. Cancer Epid, Biomarkers and Prev 2009;18:1-9), (Wu AH, Am J Clin Nutr 2009).

This is obviously a significant positive finding in regards to consuming soy.

Doctors have traditionally recommended post-menopausal women, as well as women with a history of breast cancer and those who are taking estrogen receptor modulator drugs (such as Tamoxifen™), to avoid soy all together, as it competitively binds to the same estrogen receptors sites that bind to these anti-cancer medications. However newer studies challenge the assumption that soy may be harmful in this population of women with breast cancer. A recent study published in 2009 found that, among Chinese women with breast cancer, soy food consumption was significantly associated with decreased risk of death and recurrence (Shu XO, Zheng Y, Cai H, Gu K, Chen Z, Zheng W, Lu W. Soy food intake and breast cancer survival. JAMA: 302(22):2437-43 Dec, 2009).

As the more recent, newer literature states, the probability of soy being harmful to those with breast cancer may be small or non-existent. This is an on-going, active area of study.

My recommendation would be for any interested individual to search the Internet for scientific articles and studies. Keep your search to reputable, well-established academic websites. Become familiar and informed and then speak with your physician, cancer or integrative medicine specialist, or a registered dietician, about the use of soy, in regards to your particular situation or inquiry.

The bad

The downside of soy is that although soy contains healthy omega 3, it also contains a large amount of omega 6. For example 100 grams of soybean oil contains 7 grams of omega 3 and 51 grams of omega 6 (wikipedia.com).

While we need both of these fatty acids, (with slightly more omega 6 than omega 3), the fast food type diets we consume today that are highly processed, fried and chemically enhanced, contain way too much omega 6.

The take home message should be that soy is safe and a great source of protein that has no saturated fat and is loaded with beneficial nutrients. It should be consumed in moderation and be included as part of a healthy inflammation reducing type diet, because the benefits outweigh the risks.

Soybeans, tofu, tempeh and soy milk are four great sources of soy protein that may help to reduce levels of pain and inflammation.

Therefore, in moderate amounts, soy consumption is recommended as an affordable alternative source of protein.

It needs to also be mentioned that just like with cow milk, peanuts and other foods, there may be some individuals who may be allergic to soy. Initial sampling in small quantities is recommended.

According to the USDA, 10% to 35% of the calories we consume should come from a protein source. Always try to choose lean protein and limit the fat content.

Proteins provide 4 kilocalories per gram of energy. Proteins are present in all living matter.

Proteins typically make us feel fuller after we consume them, giving them the highest satiety index. What this means is that protein tends to fill us up faster and as a result, we tend to eat less and consume less calories.

Many weight loss diets have been based on meals composed of high protein content. While these types of high protein diets do result in weight reduction, their long-term health effects if any, are as yet unknown and contradictory.

For example, protein is needed for adequate bone formation. Some studies, however, have linked the excessive consumption of high protein foods with the development of osteoporosis, due to increased excretion of calcium in the urine. Other studies however, have not demonstrated any such association.

Individuals with renal insufficiency, renal failure or pre-dialysis should be careful with their amount of protein intake, as renal function worsens and can cause toxicity in these patients. People who suffer from ulcerative colitis should avoid red meats, sausages, eggs, fats and fried foods, because they have difficulty in removing hydrogen sulfide, (a bi-product of protein breakdown that tends to accumulate in the intestinal lumen, causing even more gastric discomfort and potential complications).

Processed meats

Processed meats include our traditional favorites such as hot dogs, bacon, sausage, pepperoni, lunchmeats and canned meats. They are processed because they have a chemical agent called sodium nitrite. It is added to these meats as a color enhancer and preservative in order to control bacterial growth.

Any meat product that has been altered for flavor or convenience falls into the processed meat category, which pretty much means just about everything many of us have grown up eating. Sodium nitrite is not added to fish or chicken products.

Nitrites are dangerous because they can be converted in the stomach to nitrosamines, which are known carcinogens.

High consumption of processed meats is associated with increased incidence of esophageal, lung and gastric cancers. This is because nitrites can undergo further toxic conversions and turn into pro-cancerous reactive substrates.

A 2005 University of Hawaii study found that <u>processed meats increase the risk of pancreatic cancer by 67 percent.</u>

Some investigators have even labeled processed meats as too dangerous for human consumption.

Additional recommended reading about processed meat is the article: Nitrate, Bacteria and Human Health, in Nature Reviews Microbiology 2, 593-602 (July 2004).

Cured meats

Cured meats are those that are preserved with salt, sugar, nitrates, nitrites and smoking. These are all techniques and methods applied to meats to preserve them and add flavor. These chemicals can cause direct damage to the gastric mucosa, and consumption of cured meats have been associated with gastric cancer (Key TJ, Schatzkin A, Willett WC, Allen NE, Spencer EA, Travis RC. Diet, nutrition and the prevention of cancer. Public health nutrition 7(1A):187-200 Feb, 2004).

Charred meats

When meats are cooked at high temperatures, or are burnt, as can typically occur while cooking on an open fire, barbecue, as well as when we grill or fry them, substances called heterocyclic amines are produced. These are compounds that damage cellular DNA and contribute in the development of gastric and colorectal cancers.

So it is a good idea to try to cook your meats as well done as you enjoy them, without burning them too much.

((disclaimer))

I hope that no one jumps to the conclusion and seriously thinks that I am an alarmist, I avoid eating meats and am encouraging you to eat only twigs. This is not the case. While I do eat meat, I also admire and respect those who don't eat meat. In fact, during the research for this book, I came across a lot of research and scientific papers that indicates that vegetarians and those who stay away from eating meat on a regular basis, tend to be healthier than carnivores.

My intent is only to empower, inform and educate you so that you may have some knowledge about food. Ultimately, it is up to you to make educated decision as to what foods are nutritionally best for you and your family.

2. Carbohydrates

Carbohydrates comprise the second group of macronutrients.

Carbohydrates are substances composed of simple sugars. They come in different forms and compositions and include sugars, starches and dietary fibers.

Carbohydrates come is a wide range and are of different varieties, many of which seem to be unrelated to each other and seemingly appear to have nothing in common.

Carbohydrates include soda, candy, artificial syrups, sugar, white rice, white bread, potatoes, white pasta, desserts, milk, yogurt, fruits, vegetables, brown rice, oats, cooked grains, natural cereals, hard grainy breads, sweet potatoes (with skin) and many other substances that break down into sugars. As illustrated by this list, a wide and diverse range of food items.

The first nine items mentioned above are carbohydrates of poor nutritional quality that contributes to weight gain and obesity. They should be avoided as much as possible. The remaining carbohydrates are considered better choices that we should try to consume when possible.

Carbohydrates are our principle dietary energy source. They are a cheap source of fuel, as they are found in virtually any plant. Depending on the country, the level of economic or financial resources available, the accessibility or mobility of the population and the culture, carbohydrates tend to be the main source of food in the diets of most people. Like proteins, carbohydrates provide 4 kilocalories per gram of energy. They provide between 50-65% of the total caloric intake for humans across the world. This makes carbohydrates the most consumed macronutrient around the world.

Carbohydrates can be classified in several ways.

They can be classified as soluble or digestible (starches and sugars), and insoluble or indigestible (as is the case with fiber).

Another classification divides carbohydrates into groups according to the number of individual simple sugar units they are composed of. This classification gives us monosaccharides, disaccharides, and polysaccharides. Polysaccharides are further classified as complex or simple.

Some of the most frequently consumed monosaccharide carbohydrates in our diet include glucose (dextrose), fructose (levulose) and galactose.

These six-carbon sugars (that will be explained in greater detail shortly) are known as monosaccharides because they are single sugar molecules. Biologically, they form the simplest sugar unit.

By combining two monosaccharide or simple sugar molecules together, a longer carbohydrate molecule, called a disaccharide, is formed.

Disaccharides include 1) lactose, which is the sugar found in milk and dairy products. It is formed by the combination of glucose with galactose; 2) maltose, which is formed by the combination of 2 glucose molecules; 3) sucrose (cane sugar), which is formed by the combination of a glucose molecule and a fructose molecule; and 4) lactulose, which is formed by the combination of a fructose molecule and a galactose molecule.

People with lactase deficiency cannot digest this component of the milk and soon develop intolerance to dairy products.

Interestingly, adults who can digest and tolerate dairy products and are considered lactose tolerant, are able to tolerant dairy because of a genetic mutation. This is because gene responsible for encoding lactase activity is typically only active during infancy and slowly deactivates, as we get older.

Oligosaccharides are carbohydrates that contain 3 to 10 simple sugars linked together. When it comes to our health these molecules have gained special attention because of the difficulty in breaking these down in our digestive system. Because of this, these substances are able to reach the colon, pretty much intact and undigested (much like fiber), allowing the growth of certain strains of good bacteria. Thus, oligosaccharides serve to allow the growth of healthy colonic bacteria, which are given the name of prebiotics.

Prebiotics are defined as non-digestible food ingredients that stimulate the growth and/or activity of bacteria in the digestive system, that are beneficial to human health.

This differs from probiotics, which are "live" microorganisms that are ingested.

The end result of both of these compounds is an increase in the numbers of lactic acid bacteria (lactobacilli) as well as bifidobacteria—2 of the most common types of health promoting digestive bacteria.

Polysaccharides are carbohydrates arranged in a straight or linear arrangement, composed by monosaccharides and disaccharides.

Another attempt at classifying carbohydrates comes in the form of categorizing them as simple or complex carbohydrates.

Simple carbohydrates is a term given to structures composed primarily of monosaccharides and disaccharides, whereas complex carbohydrates are structures composed of longer sugar molecules or polysaccharides.

These classifications are confusing and are typically avoided as foods may sometimes belong to or have components of both. These are also structural classifications that pertain to the sugar molecule.

A better way to describe and classify carbohydrates is by their functional effects.

The functional effect of a carbohydrate allows us to get a better understanding of the difference between the good carbohydrates and bad carbohydrates.

This is what is important for us to keep in mind when choosing a healthy diet. It is also worthwhile to note that all carbohydrates, regardless of their complexity or molecular structure, are only absorbed in their basic monosaccharide form.

Also remember that regardless of how a carbohydrate is classified or what category we lump them into, all carbohydrates are simply molecules of sugar of varying lengths.

Now, here's the basic lowdown on understanding how carbohydrates are broken down and digested and I'm going to try and keep it simple.

Insulin is a hormone secreted by the pancreas in response to circulating blood sugar levels. The major function of insulin is in regulating the body's carbohydrate and fat metabolism and in countering the action of hyperglycemia-generating hormones. Insulin moves the circulating blood sugar into the cells where it is stored.

There are other regulatory hormones and chemical mediators secreted in response to a carbohydrate meal, but insulin is the most important one.

When we consume a meal containing carbohydrates, this macronutrient is broken down into its basic glucose components. These components then either enter the blood stream, where it results in elevated glucose levels and an appropriate insulin response, or it is stored as glycogen in the liver and the muscles. Once all the glycogen stores are full, any continued carbohydrate ingestion will result in fatty acid synthesis (production). The excess glucose is turned into fat and stored for use at a later time.

With continued carbohydrates consumption, our pancreas will reach a point when it simply cannot keep up with the continuous elevated circulating blood glucose levels and insulin resistance occurs. Levels of insulin resistance are frequently found in overweight and obese individuals. Because of this insulin resistance, we may eventually need to take oral diabetic medications to help stimulate the pancreas. (Insulin resistance is also the principal reason why some people are able to stop or reduce their oral hypoglycemic medications after weight loss is achieved through exercise and better nutrition).

Children and young adults especially, may even need administration of exogenous insulin, as insulin resistance progresses and the pancreas continues to shut down, no longer able to meet the insulin demands of the body.

In the absence of insulin, the cells of the liver, the muscles and fat tissue cannot utilize the glucose. Instead, fats from the body's fat stores are used as an energy source. (Over time, this process in individuals with insulin dependant diabetes produces a series of metabolic effects that results in increasing blood sugar levels, weight loss, frequent urination, dehydration, weakness, and the development of circulating fat breakdown chemicals called ketones. If the condition is left uncontrolled and untreated, it can lead to death).

Now lets consider the opposite effects. By increasing the amount of insulin we administer, or by simply reducing the amount of carbohydrates we eat, our body will eventually begin to use up its stores of glycogen as its source of energy. As a result, the blood sugar levels will in time, start to decline.

By increasing utilization of glycogen, as occurs with exercise or a reduction in carbohydrate intake, sugar levels will continue to decline and stabilize. As a result, secretion of insulin will also decline, producing a beneficial effect.

This process, in which the body changes its energy source from stored carbohydrates (in the form of glycogen) to instead using up and burning fat for energy, is called nutritional ketosis. It is one of the processes responsible for the weight loss seen in low—carb diets.

Good carbs, bad carbs.

Depending on the type or quality of the particular carbohydrate we consume, the pancreas will secrete insulin in order to maintain the circulating blood sugar levels under control. This occurs in either rapid, short bursts or in a steady, continuous fashion, depending on the rate in which the sugars are broken down.

When we consume poor quality carbohydrates, such as table sugar, white breads, soda and other food items composed of processed and refined simple sugars, our blood glucose levels will spike quickly after we consume them. Carbohydrate food substances such as long, starchy grains or puffed food items that have large surface areas will also result in a large amount of sugar molecules and a resulting spike in insulin secretion.

This occurs because carbohydrates of poor quality are simple structures that are easily broken down by our gastric enzymes. They are released into the blood stream in quick bursts, creating irregular peaks and valleys of blood sugar levels. When there is a blood sugar rise or peak, insulin is secreted in a similar fashion in order to reduce the glucose load.

When blood glucose levels start to decrease, we start to feel hungry.

This decrease in circulating sugar level, or hypoglycemia, acts as a trigger to stimulate our appetite to correct the low glucose levels. A low blood glucose level is the main stimulus for our hunger center in the hypothalamus. As a result, we eat.

The most common types of carbohydrates we have been consuming in increasing amounts happen to be poor quality carbs that cause these pro-inflammatory peaks and valleys in insulin secretion.

Soft drinks have replaced water, french fries have replaced salads and candy bars and other sweets have replaced fruits. A pattern of eating sugary, unhealthy high caloric foods that briefly fills us up and leads to a cycle of increase hunger and increased eating.

This pattern is typical of our unhealthy, fast food, Western diet, which we have been consuming for years. A diet and nutrition pattern, which has been an important cause for our levels of obesity and obesity related illnesses.

Physiologically, the end result is insulin that is being secreted in frequent bursts in order to regulate and control the erratic sugar elevations, which are commonly caused by poor quality carbohydrates that comprise unhealthy diets.

This produces a vicious cycle in which our bodies are continuously trying to balance and maintain a normal (euglycemic) or steady glucose level. It is the irregularity of the glucose levels with its highs and lows and the subsequent matching insulin secretion to correct it that causes hunger and inflammation. This <u>inflammation is caused by increased glycation, fatty acids and pro-inflammatory eicosanoids, (all chemicals that are produced in our bodies in the process of breaking down foods</u>). Macrophages, the previously mentioned white blood cells, are also thought to play an important immunologic role. They do so, by releasing chemical mediators called cytokins, which also contribute to the development of chronic inflammation.

The ideal carbohydrate is one that is broken down slowly and consistently. A carbohydrate molecule that is complex, and that will require time to be digested and be broken down slowly, evenly and consistently. This type of carbohydrate will result in a steady, uniform and continuous release of insulin without the bursts, peaks or valleys associated with poor quality carbs (typical of simple sugars).

This kind of carbohydrate is what is considered a good carb, and is exemplified by the carbohydrates that are found in whole grain, vegetables and fresh fruits.

Again, a wide variety of food items that seemingly appear to have nothing much in common on their surface appearance, but that share a similar make up; they are each composed of sugar molecules called carbohydrates.

The rate of carbohydrate breakdown or digestion is measured by the glycemic index and glycemic load, which will be explained shortly.

Glucose

Of all the sugars mentioned, glucose is the most important carbohydrate, because it is the favored carbohydrate utilized by most cells and tissues in the body, and is the exclusive fuel of the brain.

The role of glucose is so vital and important to the body's metabolic functions that in conditions where there are glucose shortages, the body can convert protein and fat into sugar. This process is called gluconeogenesis, which literally means "the creation of new sugar".

Another reason why it is important to know about sugar is the fact that we are consuming record quantities of it. Our consumption of sugar has been increasing steadily over the last several decades, mainly because of the high content of processed sugars that can be found in processed foods. It has been estimated that <u>individuals in the U.S. consume on average, 126 lbs of sugar a year per person, or 2-3 lbs per person, per week</u> (http://www.healingdaily.com/ detoxification-diet/sugar.htm).

This amount is not surprising, as processed sugar can be found as an ingredient listed in virtually all the nutritional labels, including many food items that don't even taste sweet.

Fructose

Fructose is the type carbohydrate or sugar that is found in fruits, vegetables and honey. We consume fructose in its natural form every time we eat natural produce. Fructose is also a great source of fiber, (another kind of healthy or good carbohydrate), that is a very beneficial digestion aid.

Natural sources of fructose include fruits, apples, pears, berries, honey, grapes and cane sugar.

High fructose corn syrup

Science and technology lead to the creation of an artificial type of sweetener derived from corn grain, called high fructose corn syrup (HFCS). The advantage of this product over table sugar was that because of the abundance and low cost of subsidized corn, HFCS could be manufactured in quantities and used as a substitute for fructose and other natural sugars. HFCS has made its way into a majority of the processed and canned food products we consume today, including countless non-sweet tasting foods that contain large amounts of carbohydrates and refined sugars. Many blame the increased, indiscriminate use of HFCS for the increase in the epidemics of obesity, diabetes and other chronic illnesses.

While every cell in the body can metabolize glucose, fructose must be broken down and metabolized in the liver.

When fructose enters the liver, the liver essentially stops working on everything else in order to metabolize the fructose. Fructose consumption results in lower levels of insulin and leptin, and higher levels of ghrelin. If you can recall from the section on fat hormones, I mentioned that leptin and insulin function to help decrease appetite. Ghrelin, (a hormone produced by the stomach and pancreas) increases appetite, which is the reason why some suspect that too much fructose consumption contributes to weight gain.

Excessive consumption of fructose, mainly in the form of HFCS, has also been blamed for the increase in cases of non-alcoholic fatty liver, as well as some cases of gout. Most importantly, it has been associated with high triglyceride levels, as well as producing levels of insulin resistance that are often indicative of pre-diabetes.

Fiber

While sugar is a type of a digestible carbohydrate, fiber is an example of an indigestible carbohydrate.

Fiber forms the indigestible carbohydrate component of plants and comes in two forms—soluble and insoluble.

The soluble portion of fiber can either be partially broken down with extreme difficulty in the digestive tract, or as it is more often, it can pass through the digestive tract in its entirety, with little or no breakdown. The soluble portion of fiber that does manage to breakdown and decompose ferments in the colon and is the substance that typically produces gas. As already mentioned, fiber functions as a pre-biotic because its slow movement through the digestive tract towards the colon allows healthy bacteria to grow and multiply.

Soluble fiber tends to bind with bile acids in the small intestine, helping to decrease levels of cholesterol.

Soluble fiber sources include prunes, raisins, plums peas, rye, chia seeds, barley, oats, berries, root vegetables, psyllium, and many others.

The insoluble portion of fiber, as the name implies, is unable to be broken down. It travels through the digestive tract intact, absorbing fluid along its transit. It bulks up and occupies more intestinal volume, which tends to produce a feeling of fullness. Cellulose, (the most abundant, natural organic compound), hemicellulose (found in bran and whole grains), and lignin's (component of the cell wall of plants) are all types of insoluble fiber. As the insoluble fiber passes through the digestive tract, it helps clear and evacuate fecal material and other digestive debris that result from the breakdown remains of ingested food substances. Insoluble fiber therefore works as a natural bowel cleaner.

Food sources of insoluble fiber include wheat, corn bran, vegetables such as celery, green beans, cauliflower, bananas, potato skins, whole grains, nuts, and seeds.

The beneficial health effects of fiber are well known. These include aiding reduce levels of colon cancer, decreasing the development of intestinal diverticula, and in providing relief from constipation and hemorrhoids. Fiber also decreases cardiovascular risks, including heart attacks by inhibiting the absorption of cholesterol and fat in the intestine (JAMA: 275 (6) :447-451). It also helps to reduce levels of elevated blood glucose by reducing the absorption of sugars from the small intestine.

Because foods with high fiber content are of a low glycemic index, they help to reduce rates of obesity by producing a steady state of insulin secretion. This in turn creates a feeling of fullness, which causes the individual to eat less.

Although fiber is recommended for as part of a healthy diet, consuming more than 50 grams a day of fiber is not recommended. Too much fiber may impede absorption of other essential nutrients as well as interfere with the absorption of medications.

Much of the research that has been published indicates that simple or the bad carbs are the main culprit responsible for most of society's health issues. Many weight loss diets have even removed all carbohydrates from their diets. As we can all recognize by now, this is a simple and foolish approach.

Just as there are different sources of protein, some which are healthier and more beneficial than others, there are also differences in the types of carbohydrates we can choose to consume.

Let's skip all the confusion and misleading information about avoiding this particular macronutrient altogether from our diet and recognize that your body needs to consume carbohydrates, as it does proteins and fats. The important thing to remember is to eat the right kinds of carbohydrates and the right amounts.

All weight loss diets that eliminate carbohydrates from the diet (an elimination diet), will produce initial weight loss because of the ketosis effect that results by the breaking down protein and fat stores. This leads to water and fluid loss, muscle loss and as a result weight loss.

Muscle tissue and muscle mass, utilizes and burns more calories (this is one reason why training with weights is recommended). Eventually, an unchecked and continued low carbohydrate diet will result decreased muscle mass. In turn, your body's metabolism will slow down.

Sooner or later your body will start to crave and seek out carbs. As you reintroduce them into your diet, the entire cycle of bursts of insulin secretion begins, and this results in increasing hunger and more insulin secretions. A cycle that in turn will eventually lead to weight gain that is more excessive than your original weight.

The USDA recommends that a non-diabetic person of normal weight, obtain 45 to 65% of their daily calories from carbohydrates.

Carbohydrates are necessary for the formation of coenzymes and DNA. They are required for normal function of the brain, heart, kidneys, the muscles of the body and the intestinal flora of the digestive tract.

As previously mentioned, the intensity of the insulin response to carbohydrate load will vary depending on the quality of the carbohydrate being consumed, the amount of food intake, as well as the genetics of each individual.

Glycation reaction

Another reason why the quality of the carbohydrate we choose for consumption is important has to do with an abnormal and potentially harmful interaction that can occur between proteins or fats, with carbohydrates. These reactions can either occur inside the body (endogenous glycations), or outside, (exogenous glycations). The accumulation of the end products of these substances can cause cross-linking between carbohydrates and proteins. This is important as it may lead to substances called "advanced glycation end-products" or AGES. AGES are important in they have been associated with chronic diseases such as cardiovascular diseases, neuropathies, cancer and Alzheimer's disease. Alzheimer's disease, for example, begins with the formation of cross-linked proteins in the brain and eventually other sticky protein deposits called amyloid deposits. This is another indication of why some people who suffer from dementia or mild Alzheimer's disease may benefit from a change in their diet.

In addition to damaging and altering the cellular structures of the individual tissues affected, these AGES also release hydrogen peroxide as a by-product of their interaction. This substance is very damaging to the tissues.

Another product of glycation reactions is glycated hemoglobin (also known as glycosylated hemoglobin or HbA1c). This reaction occurs when hemoglobin is exposed to circulating levels of glucose and allows for routine assessment of glucose control in diabetics.

Diabetics are also more likely to develop cataracts, which is another form of cross-linked protein deposits in the lens of the eye.

Diabetics are not the only individuals who suffer from the effects and consequences of glycation reactions. People who eat too many carbohydrates, or eat carbohydrates of poor nutritional quality, are prone to frequently develop advanced glycation end products. This is because they have more recurrent episodes of elevated blood glucose levels, which is what is needed for these reactions to develop.

AGES are pro-inflammatory.

They increase levels of systemic inflammation and facilitating the development of chronic illness.

It is worth repeating that carbohydrates should not be excluded from the diet. Rather, what is critically important is that we consume the right kinds of carbohydrates (this is especially true for diabetics).

The selection and consumption of healthier carbohydrates, like the selection and consumption of lean protein and healthy fats, not their elimination, forms the basis of anti-inflammatory type of diet.

What we want to recognize and do is reduce and eliminate foods that are pro-inflammatory and lead to a state of chronic inflammation. Instead we want to eat healthier food choices from all three of the macronutrient groups that are high in flavor, taste, and nutrition, and contain natural anti-inflammatory anti-oxidants.

Two terms have been created that allow identification of healthier, beneficial carbohydrates. They are: glycemic index and glycemic load.

Foods with a low glycemic value help maintain a physiologic or normal control of sugar metabolism and insulin secretion. They can improve the effect of endogenous insulin produced by the body.

Glycemic index

The glycemic index was created as a way for people to have a way to compare the different carbohydrates. As previously mentioned, each carbohydrate will differ in its sugar type and sugar content. The glycemic index ranks foods numerically from 1 to 100 depending on the intensity with which the blood sugar rises after its ingestion of a particular carbohydrate. This number is compared to a "standard," such as the glucose elevation response that occurs after eating a slice of white bread.

The glycemic index only tells us how fast a carbohydrate is turned into sugar.

The quality of a carbohydrate, as well as the content or presence of fiber in the particular food, will also influence the glycemic index.

The higher the glycemic index number, the faster and easier it will be to digest and break down the carbohydrate. As a result, there will be higher levels of circulating blood sugars and the resulting cycle of insulin bursts will also be greater. Therefore, the higher the glycemic index number associated with the carbohydrate, the worse the carbohydrate.

Food products with a low glycemic index are those between 1 and 55, intermediate range are those between 56-69 and food items with a high glycemic index are between 70 and 99. For comparison, the glycemic index of table sugar is 100. Typically, the good carbohydrates are found in the lower end of the glycemic index.

Low glycemic index foods are comprised of compact and dense components, causing them to be digested slowly. As a result of this slow, continuous and more complete digestion, the resulting sugar molecules produced will also be at a steady rate and level. This allows insulin to be secreted accordingly. There is no spiking of insulin secretion; rather, a continuous level of insulin is produced, which is the ideal insulin secretory pattern.

Some foods with a low glycemic index include grains like barley, quinoa, brown rice, black rice, rye, oats, whole wheat, spaghetti, tortillas, and wheat bread or breads made from grains.

Long grain white rice, like basamati, arborio risotto, doongara, or moolgari type rice, have a lower glycemic index as opposed to the jasmine type of white rice. The difference in the glycemic index between white rice has to due with its starch content and starch quality.

Fresh fruit, (which does not include the canned or processed fruits with added sugars) such as apples, apricots, cherries, grapefruit, grapes, oranges, peaches, plums, prunes and pears also have a low glycemic index.

Vegetables like raw carrots, sweet potatoes and peas. Beans; black beans, white beans, garbanzo beans, lentils and soy. Peanuts and yogurt are also some other foods of low glycemic index.

Regular cow milk that has a high saturated fat content has a lower glycemic index (GI: 11-40) than skim milk (GI :25-48).

This is just a partial list. For more information there are numerous books on the subject as well as on-line websites including: www.glycemicindex.com.

Benefits of low glycemic index foods include: maintaining prolonged physical energy levels, reducing the risk of cardiovascular diseases and visual disorders, reducing the development of type 2 diabetes, increasing good cholesterol (HDL), while reducing bad cholesterol (LDL) and triglyceride levels, maintaining more stable circulating insulin levels, and helping you feel fullness faster, which reduces the amount of food we eat.

More importantly, low glycemic foods prevents formation of pro-inflammatory substances.

What we must do is learn to identify and choose foods with low glycemic index because they produce a more gradual and sustained elevation of circulating blood glucose and insulin levels, which more closely resembles the normal physiological response.

By contrast, foods with high glycemic index are those that are digested and broken down quickly with a resulting increase and spike in the blood sugar levels that will require a similar, non-physiologic and marked secretion of insulin.

Examples of food items with a high glycemic index as you can guess, are those that are broken down quickly and erratically. These include white bread, corn chips, cornflakes, sodas, artificial sweeteners, white potato, mashed potatoes, fries, instant rice, white rice, cookies, donuts, cereal, watermelon and other products that contain high amounts of refined sugars.

Glycemic load.
Unlike the glycemic index, which gives a general number classification for food based solely on speed with which it increases the level of circulating blood sugar, the glycemic load

gives us the amount of carbohydrate that is contained in the particular food serving.

Both the glycemic index and glycemic load gives are useful in giving us a better understanding and more complete picture of the effect of the carbohydrate on our blood glucose level.

The glycemic load indicates the rate at which a particular type of carbohydrate is converted into sugar, taking into account the amount of carbohydrates that is contained in the food (which will depend on the portion size).

Glycemic load = glycemic index multiplied by the carbohydrate content of the food, divided by 100.

Just like the glycemic index is based on numbers, so too is the glycemic load.

A low glycemic load food is given a value between 1 and 10, an intermediate glycemic load food is valued between 11-19, and high glycemic load food is assigned a value above 20.

For example, a slice of watermelon contains a high glycemic index of 72. However, the carbohydrate content of the melon is only 5%, as the majority of the slice of melon is made up of water.

Since we know that the slice of watermelon is composed of only 5% carbohydrate, the glycemic load for a slice of watermelon is expected to be low, and in fact it is, calculated at 3.5.

A slice of white bread contains a high glycemic index of 95, meaning that it will cause our blood sugar levels to spike and rise very quickly. The carbohydrate content of the slice is 50% (in this case, it is higher than that of the watermelon); therefore, because of the higher amount of carbohydrate content, it results in a higher glycemic load of 48.

Low glycemic load foods consist of fruits and vegetables that are high in fiber, like bran cereals and beans. High glycemic load foods include (again), white potatoes, soft drinks, and processed breakfast cereals to name just a few. Mediterranean and anti-inflammatory type diets typically have a low glycemic index and glycemic load patterns.

These terms are useful, and are mentioned as additional tools you should recognize. My goal is to share with you concepts you can use to make better food choices.

Do not to allow yourself to get confused or frustrated if you do not clearly understanding these concepts right away. I too found them initially confusing, as well.

Glycemic index and glycemic load are frequently mentioned today in association with nutritional topics, which is why they are important to mention. I encourage everyone to continue reading about them until you feel comfortable what they represent.

3. Fats

Finally, we arrive at the third class of macronutrients: fats.

Fat intake is important because although we don't deliberately sit down to eat a plate of fat at our meals, we are consuming greater amounts of animal proteins that contain fat, as well as consuming greater amounts of processed snacks and fried foods that have been exposed to some form of fat.

Fat is defined as a substance that is soluble in organic solvents but not in water. So much for that definition!

According to the USDA, 20-30% of the calories we consume should come from fat.

Like carbohydrates, there are many ways to define or categorize dietary fat. It can get quite technical and complicated, which is why I will attempt to make it as relevant and as easy as possible to understand.

At room temperature, fats can be found in either a solid form such as lard (animal fat), butter and margarine (hydrogenised vegetable oils), or in liquid form such as we find with the different types of oils.

The difference between fat and oil has to do with the individual melting or boiling point temperature of each individual substance.

Natural fats come in 3 forms, all of which contain the same basic frame. They all have a backbone structure composed of a molecule of glycerol and 3 molecules of a fatty acid. A fatty acid molecule in turn, is composed of an organic acid that contains a carboxyl group attached to a carbon chain (this is keeping it simple!). These fatty acid components are connected together via attachments called bonds, which can be either a single connection between the atoms or a double connection.

It is the absence or presence of these double bonds (double connections) in the particular fatty acid that result in the classification of saturated or unsaturated fatty acids.

These compounds are also classified according to their varying sizes—from short chain to long chain fatty acids (hope you are still with me).

Based on the above explanation, we obtain three natural forms of fats that are classified as saturated fat, monounsaturated fat, and polyunsaturated fat.

Saturated fats are long fatty acid chains that don't have double bonds between the carbon atoms. They also contain a maximum number of hydrogen atoms bonded to each carbon. That is how the name "saturated" came to be. Saturated fat sources typically come from animal products and have been frequently regarded as being a type of bad fat that should be avoided, because they have been linked to deleterious health issues. These health issues include raising cholesterol levels, increased levels of breast cancer (Boyd NF et al November 2000, British Journal of Cancer 62 (9): 1672-1685), ovarian cancer (Huncharek M, Kupelnick B (2001) Nutrition and Cancer 40 (2): 87-91), and colorectal cancer (Food, Nutrition, Physical Activity and the Prevention of Cancer: a Global Perspective), as well as liver dysfunction (Mahfouz M (1981). Acta biologica et medica germanica 40 (12): 1699-1705), and depression.

Both saturated and trans fats have been linked with Alzheimer's disease (Morris MC et al. (February 2003). "Dietary fats and the risk of incident Alzheimer disease". Arch Neurol 60 (2): 194-200).

Saturated fats are easier to burn and be used as fuel but in our typical Western diet, we consume too much of it. Like saturated fats, polyunsaturated fats are chemically unstable and are easily susceptible to breakdown and oxidation by heat, light and other processes that can result in damaging and toxic, oxidation end products (which are also pro-inflammatory).

Examples of saturated fats include dairy products like cheeses and cream, coconut oils, butter, palm oil, and the fats contained in meat. Baked goods, like cakes, pastries, candies especially sweet chocolate, and processed foods are also sources high in saturated fat.

Unsaturated fats typically come from plant sources and contain at least one double bond in its structure. Monounsaturated fat has one double bond and polyunsaturated fats contain more than one.

Differing from the saturated fatty acids, these fatty acids are unsaturated because the presence of the double bond prevents a hydrogen atom from bonding and occupying all positions. Thus, the structure is not loaded with this atom (hence unsaturated).

Sources of healthy unsaturated fats include nuts (preferably unprocessed nuts) such as walnuts, cashews, almonds and pistachios, flax seed, olive oil, canola oil, and avocados to name a few.

Trans fats are typically fatty acids that contain a double bond. This means it starts off with an unsaturated fatty acid molecule, to which hydrogen is added at a high temperature, converting it into a partially or completely saturated fat. The addition of this extra hydrogen occurs in a position opposite the normal structure, giving rise to the name of trans fat.

Trans means, in opposite arrangement or on the opposite side. The trans-configuration of this fatty molecule causes these fats to be more tightly compacted, which allows for greater heat resistance. This has added value in the fast food and restaurant industry, as cooking oils can be re-utilized and last longer before having to be discarded.

The hydrogenation process allowed for the economical conversion of liquid oils into a solid form. It also stabilized the oils so that they would not freeze, be metabolized or degraded like other oils. This allows them to last longer and be reused for prolonged periods.

Another advantage of hydrogenation of fats is that it also provided unique qualities to margarine, which allows for it to be taken out of cold storage and spread on food without the need to wait and thaw to become soft and spreadable. It also provided for better baking characteristics.

Partial hydrogenation is routinely used in baked goods, fried foods and snack foods. This is mainly because it increases the shelf life of the food product and avoids the need for refrigeration. These hydrogenated fats have replaced natural fats within the processed food industry.

A natural type of trans fat can be found in small amounts in the beef of cattle as well as certain animal milks. At one time, these were the only kinds of trans fats consumed by people.

The use and production of hydrogenated fats (trans-fats) and partially hydrogenated vegetable oils have been around for over 100 years, but their use has continued to steadily increase over the last 40-50 years. Currently, it is used almost exclusively in the baking industry.

Margarine, partially hydrogenated oils and corn oil should be used sparingly.

Trans fats are unhealthy because they raise bad cholesterol (LDL) and lower the good cholesterol (HDL). An article from 1994 estimated that trans fats caused annual 20,000 deaths by heart disease in the U.S. (Willett WC, Ascherio. American Journal of Public Health 85 (3): 411),

This number of cardiac deaths attributable to trans fat was later increased in 2006, to between 30,000 and 100,000 (Mozaffarian D, Katan MB, Ascherio A, Stampfer MJ, Willett WC (2006). N. Engl. J. Med. 354 (15): 1601-13).

The incidence of cardiovascular disease and myocardial infarction (MI) started increasing and reached its peak by the 1970's. An increasing amount of evidence revealed an association between atherosclerosis (hardening of the arteries) and saturated fat consumption in comparison to the low number of heart attacks seen in European countries during WWII when such fats were in short supply. This association was described based on the rising numbers of men suffering heart disease, occurring as a result of increased prosperity that allowed for the increased consumption of meats, butter and other animal food products (Malmros, 1980).

Of all the macronutrients, fat provides the highest source of energy, at 9 kcal per gram, which is more than twice the caloric load in comparison to the 4 kcal per gram for both protein and carbohydrate.

Fat is the substance that adds flavor to meals and gives it texture and consistency.

Cuts of beef will vary depending on what part of the animal the particular cut comes from, as well as its fat content.

Fat is what makes a burger juicy and tender. Unfortunately, fats don't make us feel full as fast or much as the other macronutrients. Consequently, people who consume fatty foods or meals tend to eat more than those eating carbohydrate or protein meals. Dietary fats can come from plant or animal sources.

Fats, like carbohydrates, have also been singled out and associated with being bad for our health. It has been suggested that fat is a macronutrient that should be avoid at all costs, as was the case during the reduced-fat, fat free fad craze of the 1990's.

But we now know that not all fats are created alike and that the real danger lies in saturated fats, the trans fats commonly used in food preparation and partially hydrogenated fats found in snack foods. All are types of fats that are pro-inflammatory.

The increased health concerns and related health care costs associated to the increased fat consumption (especially attributed to trans fat use) caused New York City to became the first major U.S. metropolitan area to pass regulation, banning restaurants and food establishments from selling foods prepared with trans fat.

The bad reputation attributed to certain types of fat came about as a result of our increased consumption of processed foods and snacks that contained and were produced with saturated and/or trans fats, as well as the increase consumption of high caloric fried foods. Both factors which are typical of our economical, accessible, nutrient poor Western style diet.

We are simply eating way too much of the bad fats.

There is also research that indicates that in some individuals fats can be addictive, making their brains crave it and consume it without being able to feel full.

The truth is, however, that fats are needed in our diet as they have a multitude of beneficial health and biochemical effects.

Now that I have mentioned many negative associations, let me mention some good aspects of dietary fats.

First of all, as already mentioned, fat is our main source of energy and triglycerides (a form of circulating fat) are the main source of our dietary fat energy.

In times of famine or nutritional need, our body's fat stores can be broken down and converted into glucose as was previously mentioned.

Fat is also needed to appropriately utilize many important fat-soluble vitamins such as vitamin A, D, E and K.

Fats are used in the making of hormones, including adrenal hormones that regulate our metabolism and sex hormones, as well as substances called prostaglandins. These substances have a multitude of functions ranging from helping with calcium absorption, to protecting against cell damage, regulating blood pressure and body water balance.

Cholesterol is a type of fat that is found exclusively in animal sources. In the body it is an important fat substance that is used to produce hormones and bile acids as well as to maintain the stability of the membranes of the cells.

We acquire cholesterol from external animal fats like dairy products, beef, shrimp and pork, and we can also make our own. The liver is the main site of cholesterol synthesis within the body, responsible for 25% of the body's cholesterol production. The liver is also the primary site of fatty acid synthesis.

Fat from excessive fat consumption is stored as triglycerides in fat (adipose) tissue.

As mentioned previously, fatty acids are joined together and give rise to monounsaturated, polyunsaturated and saturated fats. There are also other fatty acids called "essential fatty acids" that includes the omega fatty acids that we will now mention.

Essential fatty acids are fatty acids needed by the body for a variety of biologic and physiologic functions. They cannot be synthesized or produced and therefore must be acquired through the diet. There are 2 essential fatty acids: alpha-linoleic acid (ALA) an omega 3 fatty acid, and linoleic acid (LA), an omega 6 fatty acid.

Both of these fatty acids are types of unsaturated fats that are needed for the body's normal functioning, but each is needed in the right amounts.

These fatty acids get their name from the location of their first double bond to carbon. Omega 3 fatty acids have their first double bond in the third position, while omega 6 has a carbon-to-carbon bond at the sixth position. Again, I am not going into detail because none of us are biochemists!

Important omega 3 fatty acids include alpha-linolenic acid (ALA), eicosapentaenoic acid (EPA), and docosahexaenoic acid

(DHA). It is the latter two components of omega 3 that are synonymous with the health benefits attributed to omega 3's.

The beneficial effects of omega 3 were first described by researches studying the Inuit tribe in Greenland during the 1970's, whose diets consisted mainly of high quantities of cold-water fish. When compared to Westerners, the Inuits were found to have significantly reduced rates of cardiovascular disease. Again, it was found that diet played a significant role in this finding (Dyerberg J, Bang HO, Hjorne N (1975). Am J Clin Nutr 28 (9): 958-66).

Omega 3's are important as they function to down regulate and limit inflammation. Many of the body's own anti-inflammatory molecules are synthesized and are derived from omega 3 fatty acids.

The Seven Countries Study previously mentioned, also found a similar health benefit effect from Mediterranean type diet, which is a diet high in omega 3.

As with all countries in the Mediterranean region, olive oil formed an important and integral component of the diet, due to its abundance.

Olive oil also happens to be composed of monounsaturated fat and is high in omega 3, resulting in its multiple beneficial health effects.

Omega 3, is commonly found in cold water fish like salmon, sardines, krill, mackerel, anchovies, butterfish, herring and black cod, as well as chia, flax and hemp seeds and oil, nuts, micro-algae and kelp is a source of DHA. These food products are recommended because of the high content of omega 3 fatty acids.

The meat of traditionally raised beef cattle, and those cattle raised organically, fed their traditional grass diets, are also considered a good source of omega 3's.

This is because omega 3 fatty acids are formed in the chloroplasts of green leaves, including grasses.

Tilapia is a type of fish that has gained popularity in the U.S. because of its affordable price. Although better than fast food because it doesn't contain saturated fat, farm raised tilapia (the most commonly available variety) is low in omega 3. In fact it contains more omega 6, than omega 3, because the feed given it is corn based, which as previously mentioned, is high in omega 6.

In addition to the cardiovascular health benefits, omega 3's has been shown to be of value in reducing, alleviating and helping the following conditions: diabetes, rheumatoid arthritis, depression, dementia, asthma, macular degeneration as well as other conditions of inflammatory nature.

Elevated triglyceride levels are currently being treated in some cases with a prescription medication called Lovaza®, which is a concentrated, high dose (4gm) form of omega 3.

Omega 3 may inhibit cancer promotion as well as progression (Larsson SC, Kumlin M, Ingelman-Sundberg M, Wolk A. Dietary long-chain n-3 fatty acids for the prevention of cancer: a review of potential mechanisms. The American journal of clinical nutrition 79(6):935-45 Jun, 2004).

Possible mechanisms by which omega 3 may be protective against cancers include: suppressing production of pro-inflammatory substances called eicosanoids, reducing estrogen formation and cell growth, suppressing tumor angiogenesis as well as oxygen free radical production.

In addition to the well-recognized cardio-protective effects of omega 3, this fatty acid also plays an important role in relation to brain and mood function. In fact, 8% of the brain is composed of omega 3 fatty acids, mainly in the form of DHA.

Omega 3 is so vital for brain development and function, that eminent omega fatty acid researcher Dr. Ralph Holman of the University of Minnesota, describes DHA as being an important component in the development of the brain structure and while EPA is important for brain function.

Omega-3 supplements that are manufactured and sold in the U.S. today are of high quality, safe and free of debris. All have undergone a molecular distillation process that removes impurities such as mercury. There are supplements of Omega 3 that come in suspension (liquid), or as chewable lozenges and are available in a variety of flavors.

Adding omega-3 fatty acid supplements to your daily diet may help reduce systemic inflammation. Omega 3 supplements do not provide any significant anti-platelet effect at recommended dosage, and can be used with aspirin and blood thinners. It is frequently recommended for patients who have heart and cardiovascular disease.

The recommended daily dose of omega 3 is based on the content of EPA and DHA contained within the capsule or dose. These are the components of omega 3 that produce the most health benefits and that is recommended. In fact it A daily recommended dose of 900-1000mg of EPA/DHA is suggested.

In addition to its cardio-protective effects, this dose is also recommended to help with depressed mood.

Make sure you recognize that most omega 3 labels (or fish oil as it is also referred to) will have and show on the front label in large lettering, the total amount of fish oil per serving. What we really want to know is the amount of EPA and DHA contained in each serving. These two amounts can typically be found on the nutritional label in smaller print. Normally, the content of EPA and DHA is less than the total amount printed in big type in front of the bottle or container. The amount stated in larger print, represents the total amount of all types of fish oil contained in each serving (EPA, DHA plus other fish oils used as fillers).

I routinely recommend omega 3 supplements for my patients and take them myself.

In addition to animal sources of the omega 3 fatty acids, there are several plant sources of the healthy unsaturated omega 3 fatty acids. This is important for vegetarians and vegans to know about.

Examples of these include avocados, olive oil, canola oil, chia seeds, and pumpkin seeds, flax seeds (contains the highest concentration of all seeds and nuts), microalgae, soy, acai fruit and nuts such as walnuts, butternuts, pecans, and almonds. (In the ancient Indian medicine of Ayurveda, the almond is believed to have nutritional properties that increase intellectual status and longevity).

When choosing nuts, raw nuts and unsalted nuts are healthier and tend to last longer than most of the nuts that are roasted or processed.

Unlike most foods that are processed as a way to increase the shelf life at stores, processed and roasted nuts are less durable as they have less amount of unsaturated fat content (good fat) and are thus more susceptible to oxidation. Roasted nuts that are old or stale may have a smell similar to paint or petroleum and should not be eaten.

In addition to omega 3 content, nuts and seeds also contain high concentrations of vitamin E and fiber.

Olive oil is a basic staple of a Mediterranean type diet, which is the proto-type diet associated with reduced levels of cardiovascular disease. Again, this is because olive oil is composed of healthy omega 3 fats and natural phytochemicals (such as polyphenols) that have significant anti-oxidant properties. These properties help reduce and protect against ongoing inflammation.

Olive oil is recommended as the preferred type of fat or oil that should be used in our diet. It is so healthy, that it makes it ideal for use in frying. Its higher price, however, prevents many of us to be able to use this valuable oil to cook with.

Vegetarians or vegans who consume no animal protein must always remember to supplement their Omega 3 fatty acid intake because if they don't, they can run the risk of being deficient in this essential fatty acid.

The main sources of plant-based omega 3's include algae, chia seeds, pumpkin seeds, flax seeds, sunflower seeds and walnuts. There are also eggs and soymilk products that have been fortified with omega 3's. The oil derived from krill, a shrimp-like crustacean, is also high in omega 3's, making krill oil similar in omega 3 content, to that of salmon.

Finally, cod liver oil supplementation, is not the same as the Omega 3 fatty acids.

As with omega 3, omega 6 fatty acids are essential fatty acids because we need to obtain them from the diet. Both of these fatty acids are important for growth and development, bone health, metabolism and brain function. Unlike omega 3 fatty acids that decrease inflammation, omega 6 fatty acids tend to increase levels of inflammation.

A relationship has been established between dietary fats and insulin resistance. Many believe that insulin resistance is associated with varying levels of inflammation. In turn, this inflammation seems to be caused by alterations in the amounts of the different dietary fats we consume.

We need both omega 3 and omega 6 in our diets, with slightly more omega 6 than omega 3. However, foods that are highly processed, that are high in fat and calorie content and that are nutrient poor (typical of Western diets), contain increasingly higher amounts of omega 6. This change in the quantities or ratios of omega 6 to omega 3 consumption, has been implicated as an important factor in the production of inflammation and insulin resistance (LH Storlien; Baur, LA; Kriketos, AD; Pan, DA; Cooney, GJ; Jenkins, AB; Calvert, GD; Campbell, LV (1996). "Dietary fats and insulin action". Diabetologica 39 (6): 621-631).

The increased consumption of omega 6 has been implicated as another important factor in the development of conditions associated with high levels of chronic inflammation seen today.

Japan is a good example of this trend. Processed, franchise type fast foods similar to the ones consumed in a Western diet, have slowly emerged in their culture. What has resulted has been an increase in cardiovascular diseases, as well as the development of chronic diseases (including increased levels of obesity and diabetes) that are approaching levels similar to that seen in the United States. These increases in chronic diseases have been attributed to the high content of omega 6 fatty acids at the expense of the traditional Japanese diet, based on fish that is rich in omega 3.

Other studies from Japan are showing similar trends in the rise in Crohns disease. This is believed to be associated with an increased total intake of animal fat, as well as an increased ratio of omega 6 to omega 3 fatty acids (Shoda, 1996).

Sources of omega 6 include: vegetable oil, processed foods, refined and fried foods, soybeans, sunflower, safflower, cottonseed, egg yolks, meats, snacks foods and margarines. We are also indirectly consuming large amounts of omega 6 in the meats we consume because most animals (and farmed fish) are fed diets and feeds, composed primarily of corn and soy, both of which contain high concentrations of omega 6.

All these are factors, (the majority of which we have been unaware of), that contribute to the disproportionately excessive consumption of the pro-inflammatory omega 6's, at the expense of the healthy omega 3.

It has been suggested that humans evolved with a 1:1 ratio of omega 3 to omega 6 consumption. Today's Western diet consists of a ratio of omega 3 to omega 6 in the range of 15:1-17:1, to 14:1-25:1 (Biomed Pharmacother. 2002 Oct;56(8):365-79) and (www.umm.edu/altmed/articles/omega-6-000317.htm).

The typical American or Western diet now provides between 8-15% of omega-6 fatty acid content. Over—consumption of omega 6 fatty acids contributes to the production of chronic inflammation.

Some nutritionists have recommended an omega 6 to omega 3 ratio of 4:1, but researchers are currently studying the ideal proportions of dietary omega 6's and Omega 3's. It is believed that a reduction in consumption of Omega 6 to levels below 5% can result in a reduction in chronic inflammation levels.

In any case, the take home message is that we have been consuming a disproportionately high amount of omega 6, which is inflammatory and not enough omega 3, which reduces levels of inflammation.

Combination Omega Supplements—Warning.

Patients made me aware of combination omega capsule supplements that contain omega 3, 6 and 9. They bought these believing that more omega fatty acid means a better health benefit. Please Do Not Take these. There is no reason for omega supplements to contain anything other than omega 3. Vegans obtain omega 6 through their diets and omega 9 is a non-essential fatty acid that is produced within our body. In addition, we all now know that we are consuming dangerous amounts of omega 6 in the foods we have been eating.

For any manufacturer to produce a product that causes inflammation and potentially lead to disease is unethical, yet many reputable manufacturers continue to do so. Retailers that carry and sell these products also share the blame. (After writing to over 80 manufacturers and retailers of omega 6 supplements with my concern I received 2 responses. Each thanking me for my concern and promising to look into it.)

I also wrote the National Institutes of Health. They referred me to a Science Advisory paper published in the journal, Circulation; 2009; 119: 902-907, on omega 6 fatty acids and the risk for cardiovascular disease (http://circ.ahajournals.org/content/119/6/902.long).

After reading the paper, I contacted the principal author, omega fatty acid researcher, and Professor of Medicine, Dr. William Harris, who agreed with my concerns. Dr Harris believes that it is not so much the higher amounts of omega 6 found in our diets that is the problem, rather the insufficient amounts of omega 3 consumption that leads to disease.

Fatty acid ingestion and inflammation

Research has shown that consumption of high levels of omega 6 which are found in processed foods and meats, trigger and stimulate enzymes known as cyclooxygenase (COX) 1 and 2, that in turn produce inflammation. These are the same enzymes responsible for many inflammatory states, including arthritis. Non-steroidal anti-inflammatory medications are frequently prescribed for these inflammatory conditions, as these medications block these COX receptors in tissues, resulting in decreased inflammation and subsequent pain relief.

Again, as with any anti-inflammatory type diet, fats should not be eliminated or avoided. Rather, what we need to do is recognize and utilize the good quality, healthy monounsaturated fats from both animal and plant sources. This will provide us with a wider variety of healthy food choices, enabling us to limit and avoid the unhealthy saturated and trans-fats. In addition, I would recommend the daily supplementation of omega 3.

The Micronutrients

Micronutrients are substances that are required in small quantities by the body and are consumed in smaller amounts. Included in this category are the vitamins, minerals and trace elements. These are natural substances needed by humans and animals for normal biological functions. The human body is unable to produce these micronutrients, so they must be obtained through diet.

Important vitamins include vitamin A, B complex, B1-thiamine, B2-riboflavin, B3-niacin, B5-pantothenic acid, B6, pyridoxine, pyridoxal, B7, B8, B9, and B12 as well as vitamin C, D, E, K, biotin and carotenoids.

Important minerals include calcium, magnesium, phosphorus, chloride, potassium, sodium, iron. Important trace elements include lithium, zinc, cobalt, fluoride, manganese, molybdenum, selenium, sulfur and strontium.

Most of these substances are natural components found in foods of plant origin.

The best source of vitamins and minerals are natural fruits and vegetables. The supplements we buy at the store that come in capsule, liquid or tablet form are beneficial and recommended *as supplements*. They are nowhere near the same quality and of the variety as the vitamins and minerals found in natural foods. Plants acquired in their natural state, without being adulterated, manipulated or processed, contain a multitude of trace amounts of essential elements and compounds—many of which have not yet been synthesized. When we take pill forms of vitamin supplements, they help to ensure that we consume at least the basic required quantities of these substances. We should never believe or become accustomed to thinking however, that taking a compound created in a laboratory is equal to what we get from nature by way of fruits and vegetables.

Aside from these micronutrients, plants also contain natural antioxidant like substances known as phytonutrients or phytochemicals. (I will use both terms interchangeably throughout this book).

Phytonutrients: Nature's antioxidants

Most of us know something about vitamins and minerals or at least have heard something about them and it is not a completely foreign concept. In contrast, many of us have probably never heard the term "phytonutrients" or "phytochemicals" and for most of us it may be a new concept.

"Phyto" has Greek language roots and is the term for "plant." So that any substance that contains phyto indicates that the substance is derived from a plant source.

During the 1980s, the National Institute of Health (NIH) started conducting research to analyze various phytochemicals, to discern their preventive, protective and beneficial health effects.

This research yielded a significant amount of evidence suggesting that phytochemicals provide protection against a wide range of chronic diseases that includes cancer, cardiovascular disease, arthritis, macular degeneration, diabetes and hypertension to name a few.

Phytochemicals include many natural bioactive chemicals that include classes of substances known as flavenoids, carotenoids, phenols and polyphenols, to name a few, as there are thousands of these varying health benefiting compounds in plants.

While phytochemicals are not essential for life, they may very well play a vital, and important role to achieve optimal health, as well as in the prevention of diseases.

Phytochemicals can be considered as natures' antioxidants. <u>Antioxidants are substances that down-regulate or decrease levels of inflammation.</u>

Antioxidants are substances that destroy toxic particles known as free radicals as well as other molecules that interact with cells causing damage and altering them. These toxic substances also interfere with normal DNA production and cell growth. The end result of these chemical interactions is that cells become dysfunctional, or even worse; they can turn into cancerous cells.

<u>Free radicals occur naturally in the body, especially during the process of digestion</u>. Environmental toxins such as ultra-violet rays, chemicals, pesticides, cigarette-smoke, radiation and many other irritants can cause an increase in these molecules. Antioxidants work by reducing and preventing damage caused by these interactions. Without an adequate amount of antioxidants, oxygen metabolism may be compromised,

resulting in oxidative stress at the cellular level. Oxidative stress that in turn signals a cascade of pro-inflammatory chemicals, which trigger the inflammatory system and the development of acute and then chronic inflammation.

Chronic inflammation and oxidative stress have both been implicated as risk factors for the development of certain cancers (Coussens LM, Werb Z. Nature. 2002 Dec 19-26;420(6917):860-7). Inflammation and cancer).

The transformation from a normal cell into cancerous cells occurs throughout various steps. It has been found that some phytochemicals can interfere during various points of the cancer development process. They can either inhibit metabolic activation at the start of a cancerous transformation, suppress promotion of cancer cells, or interfere with progression towards the end of the transformation. Functions, that provide a protective barrier effect to prevent a conversion of cancer cells, or that act as blocking agents (Young-Joon Surh. Cancer chemoprevention with dietary phytochemicals. Nature Reviews Cancer 3, 768-780 (October 2003).

A phytochemical called quercetin, which is principally obtained by eating apples was shown to be inversely related with the risk of developing lung cancer. Consumption of another phytochemical called myricetin, was inversely associated with the risk of developing prostate cancer (Knekt P et. al Flavonoid intake and risk of chronic diseases. The American journal of clinical nutrition 76(3):560-8 Sep, 2002).

As previously mentioned, phytochemicals are compounds that originate from plants. The particular type of the phytochemical content and concentration will depend on the type of plant, as well as its source of origin. All types of edible food that originates from a plant source will contain these substances.

Remember also that it is from plants that we derive many of the medicines we use today. The origin of our modern pharmacopeia is derived from trees, bushes and plant sources. This is way the unique plant and flora habitats like the Amazonian jungle, must be conserved and protected from destruction.

Likewise, the extraordinary diversity of our oceans and the sea life and the marine microorganisms they contain, many of which we have yet to discover, may provide an even greater source of our future medicines and cures.

Because of the beneficial antioxidant health effects, dietary intake of phytonutrients is recommended as part of an anti-inflammatory diet. The cheapest, safest and most efficient way in which to obtain these important phytonutrients is through the foods we routinely eat.

There are many different types of phytonutrients. Some estimates put the number of these substances at well over

5000, each with specific factors and components that provide different, beneficial effects for our health.

For example, the phytochemical flavenoids, which is a class of phenolic compounds found in fruits, vegetables, chocolate and tea, can be sub-classified into anthocyanidins, flavenol (catechins), flavanones, flavones, and isoflavones.

Other phytochemicals can include many natural bioactive chemicals and include substances known as carotenoids, phenols and polyphenols, lignans, monophenols, organosulfides, phenolic acids, anthocyanins, hydroxycinnamic acids, tannins, phytosterols, stylbenes, xanthophylis, and catechins. This is just a small list, as there are hundreds of these varying phytochemical compounds found in plants.

The reason why health experts, doctors and registered dieticians recommend we include a variety of fruits and vegetables in our diet, is precisely because of the different varieties and amounts of phytonutrients found in the different types of plant based foods. Each vegetable and fruit type will contain a different variety and concentration of vitamins, minerals and phytonutrients, which are food-specific.

One way to understand this concept is by just seeing the wide range and vast assortment of colors that vegetables and fruits come in. The varying, different food colors represent the variety of phytonutrients that exist in that particular food item.

The colors of plant foods vary depending on the type and amount of phytonutrients present.

The variation in color in turn, is due to a phytochemical class called carotenoids. These are a group of fat-soluble pigments, the consumption of which has been associated with a reduction of several chronic diseases (Ziegler RG. A review of epidemiologic evidence that carotenoids reduce the risk of cancer. The Journal of nutrition 119(1):116-22 Jan, 1989).

Over 600 different kinds of carotenoid substances have already been found. The most commonly consumed by humans being lycopene, which is found in tomatoes and tomato based foods.

This is why it is recommended that you choose and eat fruits and vegetables of a variety of different colors. The pigments that give color to fruits and vegetables are the antioxidants that help down regulate inflammation and are associated with helping reduce incidences of cancers, cardiovascular disorders and other chronic diseases.

Red foods are of this color due to its content of lycopene, quercetin, and hesperidin—all of which are phytonutrients.

Lycopene is a carotenoid, whereas quercetin and hesperdin belong to the flavinoid family of phytonutrients. In addition, red foods contain anthocyanins that have been associated with reduced incidence of prostate cancer, and reducing levels of blood pressure, bad cholesterol (LDL) as well as stroke and macular degeneration.

RED foods include: cucumber, chili, peppers, strawberries, cherries, pink grapefruits, beets, tomatoes, cranberries, guavas, papayas, red apples, red onions, raspberries, red cabbage, radishes, pomegranates, watermelons and red pears.

Yellow and orange foods contain: carotenes, potassium, zeaxanthin, vitamin C, selenium, and folate. These phytonutrients help with collagen formation, promotes joint health, helps reduce cholesterol, the risk of macular degeneration and protects against prostate cancer.

YELLOW / ORANGE foods include: bananas, chayote, pineapples, grapefruits, carrots, oranges, papayas, peaches, lemons, kiwis, mangos, nectarines, apricots, cantaloupes, yellow and orange chili peppers, pears, yellow apples, yellow tomatoes, corn (maize) and yellow figs.

Green foods contain chlorophyll, fiber, leucine, vitamin C, folate, calcium and beta-carotene. These nutrients help with digestion, reduces prostate cancer, and blood pressure, bad cholesterol, maintains retinal function and acts as anti-carcinogens in the digestive tract by reducing tumor growth and inflammation.

GREEN foods include: avocado, lettuce, spinach, celery, green peppers (capsicum), broccoli, asparagus, corn, peas, green grapes, green onions, green pears, kiwis, limes, zucchini, cabbage, artichokes and leaks.

Purple and bluish colored foods contain resveratrol, vitamin C, fiber, flavonoids, ellagic acid, quercetin, and leucine. These support the immune system, provide cardiovascular protection, lower bad cholesterol and help with the absorption of calcium and minerals in the digestive tract, improving digestion and reducing certain types of cancer growth.

PURPLE and BLUE foods include: eggplant, blueberries, blackberries, raisins, grapes, plums, prunes, pomegranates and red cabbage.

Black colored foods are also very nutritious and good for you. Many of the black colored fruits and vegetables contain anthocyanins, in addition to being high in fiber, iron and vitamins.

BLACK food items include: black soy, black beans, black lentils, blackberries and black rice. Black rice is considered to be one of the healthiest, if not the healthiest, rice available. In ancient China it was valued so much, that only the emperor was allowed to eat it.

WHITE foods include plantains (bananas), white corn, white peaches, onions, cauliflower, garlic, ginger, mushrooms, shallots, and parsnips. These colored food items contain still different types of phytonutrients.

As you can imagine, this is only a partial list. You may fill in the blanks and add to this list.

In addition to vitamins, minerals, and phytonutrients, vegetables and especially fruits are also a good source of dietary fiber and water.

For a healthy diet, it is recommended that you choose green leafy vegetables, brightly colored vegetables, and lots of fresh whole fruits. You should eat at least five (preferably more) servings of fresh fruits and vegetables each day (not the canned stuff).

In a healthy, balanced, whole-food/anti-inflammatory type diet, which is the type of diet we should all be eating, variety is a key. Eating healthy is tasty and full of flavors. It tastes much better and it is better for you than the boxed pre-packaged weight loss stuff endorsed by celebrities. Once you know how to make healthy food choices, this will become the simplest, most hassle-free form of eating around.

Foods and other substances that form part of a healthy anti-inflammatory diet are selected because of their content of micronutrients.

Remember that we must all eat, so why not select foods that will work for us, instead of foods that work against us?

<u>Blood thinners and green leafy foods.</u>

As a cardiologist, I have many patients on blood thinners (anti-coagulants), specifically warfarin.

While it has been customary to tell patients to avoid green-leafy vegetables and other green colored food items while on warfarin, we now know that avoidance of these healthy foods is more detrimental than beneficial. Green leafy vegetables are healthy food choices we must all try to consume more of. They are also high in vitamin K. Vitamin K in turn alters the effect of warfarin on the blood affecting the effectiveness of the anti-coagulant treatment. This is why traditionally, the consumption of green leafy vegetables and foods has not been recommended while on anti-coagulation medicine.

Recognizing that vegetables are important as part of a healthy diet, I encourage my patients to eat them, on a case-by-case basis. When eating green foods and vegetables, what is important is to try to consume the same amounts of these foods each week. What we don't want is large shifts in food intake that will affect and alter the anti-coagulant effect. Maintaining control over portion sizes and amount, will allow for better control without wild fluctuations. There will be some situations in which eating green foods and vegetables while on blood thinners will unfortunately not be appropriate, reason for which patients on anti-coagulant treatment need to speak with their own physician before starting to eat these foods.

(In addition to green leafy vegetables and foods, soy and garbanzo beans (chickpeas) are also high in vitamin K).

Other food items with healthy and anti-inflammatory benefits.

Red Wine

Red wine is part of an anti-inflammatory diet due to its high content of natural phytochemicals, which consist of both flavonoids and non-flavenoids. Flavenoids in red wine include quercetin and rutin both of which act as antioxidants. Flavonoids are also found in other fruits such as apples and oranges, but its concentration is highest in red wine. Another component of red wine that is currently en vogue is resveratrol—an antioxidant that belongs to the non-flavenoid family of phytonutrients called "stilbenes". They are found mainly in red grapes, and wine, as well as purple grape juice. In red wines, the amount of resveratrol contained in the wine will depend on its fermentation time, as this phytochemical is found in the skin or red grapes.

Both substances, flavenoids and resveratrol, are considered to be beneficial to our health in moderate amounts, as they have been shown to increase levels of good cholesterol

(HDL), prevent microvasculature clotting (limiting blood clots), and limit inflammatory processes in the cardiovascular system. Recognition of the benefits of red wine in terms of cardiovascular health comes from multiple research studies of the French population. They consume high amounts of saturated fats, yet their rates of cardiovascular diseases are lower (the French paradox). Wine also figures prominently in the Mediterranean diet.

One, (4oz.) glass of red wine for women, and two glasses of red wine in men a day, caused a reduction in heart attacks of 30-50% (Szmitko etal, (Circulation. 2005;111:e10-e11.) © 2005 American Heart Association, Inc. This is also the amount that has been traditionally recommended by the American Heart Association.

Recently, there has been some new information that suggests that women who drank just one glass of red wine a day, increased their risk of various cancers. Although this risk was small, it was nonetheless significant to cause some experts to reconsider the accepted recommended amounts of red wine consumption for women. Until I know more, I have been recommending that women cut back and limit their red wine consumption to 3-4 glasses a week.

Chocolate / Cocoa

Cocoa contains natural polyphenol chemicals called flavan-3 ols, or flavonoids, which have been associated with a reduction in blood pressure and improving vascular endothelial function, resulting in reduced levels of inflammation. They reduce the oxidation of bad cholesterol (LDL) and decreased fasting insulin levels, which improves insulin sensitivity.

Flavenoids found in concentrated cocoa are rich in catechin and epicatechin, which are phytonutrients that are more powerful antioxidants than vitamins C and E.

For the chocolate to be effective as an anti-inflammatory agent, it must be of a high cocoa concentration—with a minimum of 70% cocoa content. In most food markets, you can now find such types of high cocoa content chocolates. Because of this high cocoa concentration, the chocolate will be bitter tasting, and its consumption will be limited to a single serving.

The sweet chocolate or the candy-type of chocolates, like a candy bar or other sweets is not the same as high cocoa chocolate, and does not count as an anti-inflammatory food item. Any chocolate item that contains sugar as the first ingredient, or has a high sugar content, will only contributes to the epidemic of obesity. Protective chocolate is pure chocolate without added sugar, milk or other added ingredients.

Tea.

There are over 3000 varieties of tea. Tea is recommended as part of a healthy anti-inflammatory diet because they contain a high content of phyto-nutrients in the flavenoid class, which includes tannins and phenolic acid.

The teas with the highest concentration of these healthy polyphenols are the natural white, green and oolong tea variety, as their phytonutrient concentrations will be found at higher levels than more processed teas.

These varieties of tea, along with black tea, are made from the leaves of the Camellia Sinensis tea plant. Green tea is the tea most associated with beneficial antioxidant effects. It is rich in a polyphenol called epigallocatechin, which has resulted to have a preventive effect against various cancers

(Yang CS, Maliakal P, Meng X. Inhibition of carcinogenesis by tea. Annual review of pharmacology and toxicology 4225-54 2002).

White teas are unprocessed, green teas are partially processed, oolongs are intermediate in terms of amount of processing, and black teas, which are the most common variety is the most processed. Therefore contains the least amounts of phyto-nutrient content.

Just like the differences between the chocolate candies versus the high concentrated cocoa chocolate previously mentioned, in order to get the full complement of phytonutrients from tea, one must consume tea that is must be made from natural tea leaves, avoiding teas that come in bottles or other containers. While these varieties may taste good, they are altered with chemicals and preservatives and are full of sugar. Some of these may even be tea-flavored soft drinks with little or no actual tea in it, so be careful and don't be fooled.

Natural healthy teas are easily recognized, as you can see the remains of the actual natural tea leaves. Most often, these come in sachets that you dissolve in boiling water to extract not only the flavors, but the nutrients as well.

The consumption of tea has been associated with a multitude of health benefits that include cardiovascular protection due to reduced LDL cholesterol and triglyceride levels, and playing a role in decreasing lipoprotein oxidation. It has been found to decrease levels of diabetes by improving insulin sensitivity, alleviating arthritic pain and inflammation, improving the immune system, alleviating digestive distress, improving cognitive function and many other beneficial health effects. Asian populations that regularly consume green tea, have lower incidences of cancer when compared to other cultures that don't drink tea as often (Siddiqui IA, Adhami VM, Saleem M, Mukhtar H. Beneficial effects of tea and its polyphenols against prostate cancer. Molecular nutrition & food research 50(2):130-43 Feb, 2006).

In addition, tea has soothing, calming, anti-spasmodic effects, which reduce high blood pressure. Green and black teas have been associated with the reduction of various types of cancers.

Tea should be consumed in moderation because many varieties contain caffeine, which may give rise to some side effects that may include restlessness and irritability. Although green tea is a substance that is generally recognized as safe, pregnant and breastfeeding women should limit their intake of tea because caffeine can be passed through the breast milk, resulting in sleep disorders in nursing infants. Individuals with peptic ulcers may also want to be cautious with their intake of green tea because it can stimulate the production of gastric acid.

Multiple studies are currently researching the beneficial health effects of tea in relation to cardiovascular diseases and cancers.

As with all anti-inflammatory food items mentioned, moderation is key.

Olive oil

Olive oil is one of natures' gifts to humanity, as it is an abundant source of the good monounsaturated fats.

Olive oil comes in a variety of forms and from a variety of places; however most of the olive oil we consume in the United States comes from countries located around the Mediterranean region (such as Italy, Greece, Spain and France). As a result, olive oil forms a basic staple of a Mediterranean type diet.

While Greece is the world's largest producer of extra-virgin olive oil, the most commonly used olive oils in the United States come from Spain and Italy.

Standards for the production of olive oils are monitored and conducted by the International Olive Oil Council based in Madrid.

It is an organization that establishes regulations and monitors the production and quality of olive oil produced from member countries.

There are different classifications of olive oils, which are based on the acidity of the oil, as well as the quality and production methods. Classification includes regular, light, virgin, extra-virgin, pure, and refined olive oil, as well as oils that are cold pressed or from the first pressing. Up until 2010, the United States Department of Agriculture, graded olive oils in grades—from grade A (superior) to grade D (substandard).

Regular olive oil is a blend of virgin and refined virgin oil containing no more than 1.5% acidity.

Light olive oil means a lighter oil color and not lower in calories or fat content. It is olive oil that results from a mixture of refined, lower quality olive oils.

Virgin olive oil has an acidity level of less than 2% and contains no refined oils. The olives used to make virgin olive oil are riper than extra-virgin oils.

Extra-virgin is oil that is obtained from the first pressing and contains less than 0.8% acidity. There are no refined or other types of oils mixed in, and is olive oil in its purest state. As such, it contains higher concentrations of the phytonutrient, polyphenol.

The healthiest olive oil is extra-virgin oil.

Consequently, it tends be the most expensive of the olive oil types.

Pure olive oil comes from the second cold pressing or chemical extraction from what is left over after the first pressing.

First press means that the oil came from the first pressing of the olive.

Pressing typically refers to the pressure applied by traditional hand presses, used to produce small amounts of oil.

Cold press means that the olive oil that results was obtained by cold methods, with no heat used during the processes. Hot water is sometimes applied to the pressing in order to extract more oil from the olive paste that results from the pressing. This is important to know, as heat can change the olive oil makeup as well as its chemistry.

Like wine, olive oil can come in a variety of colors, smells, tastes, textures and consistencies. Their characteristics will vary depending on the type of olive used, the region where the olives are grown and the climatic conditions of the region. Conditions of the soil, the temperature, humidity, rain and even the method of harvesting the individual olives, all play a crucial role in the quality of the final product.

As we all know, olive oil tends to be more expensive than other forms of oils. The purer the olive oil is, the greater the cost.

For anyone on a budget or limited resources, an economical way to purchase olive oil would be to buy it in bulk and split it with friends or family members.

It is important to remember that olive oil is essentially fruit oil. As such, we need to take special consideration when we preserve it.

We should take the same precautions to preserve olive oil as we do to preserve any fruit juice. Remember that heat, light and even air can degrade and breakdown the oil. Olive oil should be kept in small, dark colored bottles or containers and are best stored in a dark kitchen cabinets where the temperature can remain constant, and away from heat sources like the stove or oven. Refrigeration is usually not recommended because the oil can condense or even solidify, affecting the flavor. Refrigeration should not effect the composition of the oil if it is to be utilized quickly. Remember again to think of olive oil as a natural fruit juice that needs to be treated in a similar way you would a good wine.

Olive oils' anti-inflammatory properties are a result of natural chemicals called oleocanthals. These phytochemicals are more concentrated in extra-virgin oils and act like natural antioxidants by decreasing levels of inflammation (much like some of the over the counter non-steroidal anti-inflammatory medications). Oleocanthals have been shown to reduce the risk of stroke, heart disease, dementia, and some cancers linked with inflammation.

As previously mentioned, olive oil before is the principal fat used in a healthy, Mediterranean type diets, and it forms a basic component of any anti-inflammatory type diet. In addition to polyphenols, olive oil contains other antioxidants phytonutrient such as carotenoids and natural vitamin E. All of these helping lower bad cholesterol (LDL) and increase good cholesterol (HDL).

Polyhenols are found in highest concentration in extra-virgin olive oil, and include oleuropein and tyrosol, other natural anti-oxidants that protect cells against oxidative injury. Some studies have indicated that these phytonutrients are responsible for olive oils cardio-protective effects (Int J Vitam Nutr Res 75 (1): 61-70).

Olive oil consumption also helps remove excess omega 6 fatty acids, (as a result of our fast-food, processed diets), helping to regulate the balance between omega 3 and omega 6.

Clinical data has shown that regular consumption of olive oil decreases blood sugar levels and provides anti-inflammatory, anti-thrombotic and vasodilatory effects, all of which play a role in olive oils cardio-protective effects (Pharmacol. Res. 55 (3): 175-86),

Remember that although olive oil is healthy, it still remains a form of fat that is high in calories.

Besides olive oil, other healthy oils that are monounsaturated and contain omega 3's include canola oil, linseed oil, flax seed oil and hemp oil.

Anti-inflammatory Condiments

Foods are not the only edible substances that are of benefit in helping decrease and down regulate inflammation. There are also a multitude of spices with beneficial health properties, due to their unique content of anti-oxidant phytochemicals. Some of these spices include garlic, ginger, curcumin, black pepper, basil, rosemary, coriander, cinnamon, cardamom, parsley and chives.

Garlic.

Garlic has been around since the time of the Great pyramids in Egypt. Garlic cloves were valued for their medicinal properties, and given to the troops of ancient Greece and Rome during their many military campaigns. Their use in China also dates back nearly 2,000 years and can be found mentioned as a medication in the medical textbook, The Yellow Emperors Classic of Internal Medicine.

Hippocrates, who is considered the father of modern Western medicine, and Galen one of the greatest teachers of medicine, (whose names remain synonymous with the practice of medicine and physicians today), cited the use of garlic as a treatment for various medical conditions.

They described the benefits of garlic for poor digestion, respiratory disorders, fatigue and tiredness, and parasitemia.

Louise Pasteur studied garlic in the mid 1850's who was the first to notice several anti-septic and antibacterial properties of garlic. Because of this finding, garlic was used during the First and Second World Wars as an antiseptic in order to prevent wound gangrene.

Garlic is derived from varying different species. The traditional garlic we cook with today coming from the Allium Sativa species. Garlic is in the family of the onion, the shallot and chives.

Garlic is composed of many natural phytochemicals, which include allyl propyl disulphide, flavenoids, several enzymes, vitamin B, protein, minerals, saponins and others. These are natural antioxidants responsible for a multitude of beneficial health effects.

One of the chemicals isolated and studied is alliin. It's mainly alliin, which gives the smell and taste to garlic. When garlic is crushed, macerated or cut, the alliin becomes allicin—a compound that in turn contains substances related to sulfa (in the form of diallyl sulphide). These sulfa compounds are some of the phytochemicals that provide beneficial antiseptic and health effects.

Not all garlic contains the same amounts or concentrations of these healthy components, as this will depend on the origin and method of garlic harvest and preparation. That is one reason why there have been inconsistencies and differences in the published studies, looking at and trying to document health effects attributable to garlic.

Raw and aged garlic are considered the best and the most powerful types of garlic because they contain more allicin and sulfide containing compounds, which are responsible for the health benefits produced by consuming garlic.

In countries where people consume a higher amount of garlic, rates of cancers are low, raising an association between garlic consumption and rates of cancer development.

Today, garlic is used for a variety of preventive effects including for the prevention of cardiovascular disease, reduction of cholesterol levels as well as high blood pressure.

Depending on the study cited, garlic either produced reduced levels of LDL cholesterol and triglycerides or produced no significant improvement or benefit. Again, this is due to the type and quality of garlic researched in the studies.

Garlic from the Allium Sativa genus has been recognized to reduce platelet adhesion, much like the effect of aspirin. This is a potentially important finding for the treatment of coronary heart disease.

Garlic is beneficial in the treatment of diabetes, because allicin competes with insulin in the liver, freeing up insulin and causing an increase in free circulating insulin levels. It also is known to decrease levels of homocysteine (implicated in cardio-vascular disease).

It was recently found that routine intake of garlic significantly reduced markers of inflammation, which includes C-reactive protein (CRP) and homocysteine itself.

Garlic helps strengthen the immune system, helping to combat various forms of cancer. In a recent review of seven different studies, scientists reported that people who consumed high amounts of cooked or raw garlic had on average a 30% reduction in colorectal cancers.

In another study, called the Iowa Women's Health Study conducted on a group of 41,000 middle-aged women, it was shown that women who ate a diet containing fruits, vegetables and garlic had a 35% reduction in risk of developing colon cancer. It is believed that garlic may offer protection against breast cancers, prostate cancers, and cancers of the larynx.

Garlic supplements can be obtained in various forms including whole fresh garlic, dried garlic, garlic oil, or frozen garlic extract.

Ginger

Ginger is native to China and India. It has been part of traditional Chinese medicine since the beginning of its culture, as well as in Arab countries since 650 BC. It was one of the spices found on the tables of Europe along with salt and pepper. It was also one of the species used for treatment against the plague.

Ginger is commonly used to help digestion by increasing the production of gastric juices and saliva. Ginger helps to relieve abdominal pain, gas, bloating and diarrhea. It is also a good agent for gastroparesis (slow digestion), stomach cramps and constipation. Ginger increases the production of bile, which is why it is not recommended and is even contra-indicated in people who suffer from gallbladder stones. It has also been found that ginger is more effective than some anti-motion sickness drugs in alleviating vertigo and motion sickness symptoms.

Ginger works as a treatment for dizziness and nausea related to chemotherapy as well as for pregnancy—induced morning sickness. The anti-inflammatory properties of ginger help reduce muscle spasms and inflammation associated with arthritis and has mild effects in reducing cholesterol.

At the respiratory level, ginger root is used in asthma and bronchitis because it stimulates the pulmonary blood circulation. It has detoxifying effects on the body and helps cleanse the digestive tract and kidneys. Ginger produces a mild anticoagulant effect, which is why it should be used with caution in people taking anticoagulant medications.

Animal studies suggest that ginger reduces anxiety. Throughout history, ginger has also been associated with having aphrodisiac properties.

Ginger comes in various forms, including whole fresh root, dried root, ginger, crystallized ginger, pickled ginger in vinegar, as well as ginger in a preservative form.

The characteristic flavor and smell of ginger is due to a combination of oils that include gingerols, shogaols, and zingerone. It is this ginerol component that has been shown to be the most medicinally active component in ginger.

Ginger is used medicinally in different forms, depending on the region of the world used.

In India, ginger is applied as a paste on the forehead to relieve headaches, the common cold, and nausea.

In Indonesia, a ginger drink is prepared to reduce fatigue. It is also used as a supplement, given to people with decreased nutritional intake.

In Peru, pieces of ginger are dissolved in hot water and taken orally as a decoction or potion to relieve stomach pains.

In the United States ginger is approved by the FDA for the treatment of vertigo as well as pregnancy induced nausea, as well as a dietary supplement.

Ginger is currently being studied for its effectiveness against cataracts caused by diabetes and for other diabetes complications.

Turmeric

Turmeric is a species of grass that is commonly used as a dye for clothing. It is the component that gives mustard its yellow color, and is used in the traditional foods of India known as curries. It is a root that is usually boiled, dried and then ground into a powdery spice. Turmeric is related to ginger and is composed of nutritious components called curcumin, which contain potent anti-inflammatory properties. In traditional Chinese and Ayurvedic medicine, turmeric has been used to aid digestion, relieve arthritis joint pain and to regulate menstruation. It is currently used in parts of Asia as an antiseptic and antibacterial. It has also be shown that in populations that consume diets high in amounts of turmeric content have a reduced number of people who suffer from Alzheimer's disease. This may be an important finding for further research studies.

Because of its reported beneficial medicinal effects, researchers at the National Center for Complementary and Alternative Medicine are studying the anti-inflammatory effects of turmeric for a variety of diseases, including respiratory failure, liver cancer and osteoporosis.

The National Institute of Health (NIH) currently has 19 clinical trials in various stages of research.

All of these commonly used spices produce warmth and heat when consumed. As such, they have Yang characteristics. Accordingly, they are routinely used in traditional Chinese medicine beneficial for balancing conditions associated with excess cold, or Yin.

In addition to spices, there are vegetables that also contain phytochemicals and properties that help in the control of chronic inflammation and among these, are the cruciferous vegetables

Cruciferous vegetables

Cruciferous vegetables are the class of vegetables that include many of the common variety of vegetables we consume today. These include broccoli, cauliflower, cabbage, watercress, arugula, kale, collard greens, brussel sprouts, turnips, radishes and horseradish.

Cruciferous vegetables are one of the most commonly harvested plants worldwide. They are called cruciferous because of the way in which the leafy petals of these plants resemble a cross (in Latin, "crux" means "cross").

Cruciferous vegetables comprise a healthy and nutritious food group that has been found to have significant cancer modulating effects. This is due to their high content of phytonutrients called glucosinolates. When these glucosinolates are metabolized, they give rise to various other compounds that promote health. These compounds are called isothiocyanates.

Cruciferous vegetables have been found to be of benefit in reducing cancers of the bladder, breast, ovary, colon and prostate in individuals who consume cruciferous vegetables on a regular basis.

In addition to phytonutrients, cruciferous vegetables are a good source of vitamins, minerals and soluble fiber that aids in digestion.

Recent evidence from a large cohort analysis of more than 3000 breast cancer survivors showed that higher intake of cruciferous vegetables, in women taking the breast cancer medication tamoxifen, resulted in a 52% reduction in the risk for recurrent breast cancer events (Thomson CA, etal. Veg. intake asso. with reduced breast cancer recurrence in tamoxifen users. Women's Healthy Eating and Living Study. Breast cancer research & treatment Jul, 2010).

The anti-cancer properties found in cruciferous vegetables have been credited to chemicals of the isothiocynate family. These include: sulforaphane, indole-3-carbinol, di-indolylmethane and glucosinolates.

In addition, sulforaphanes have also been shown to have anti-diabetic, and anti-microbial properties.

Indole-3-carbinol is a degradation product and a result of the maceration of the vegetable fiber. It is a natural antioxidant and anti-atherogenic, that protects cellular DNA and improves DNA repair. Some studies have also shown reduced platelet aggregation (preventing sticking, like aspirin) as well as improved cholesterol and lipid metabolism.

Di-indolylmethane, is useful in improving estrogen metabolism in both men and women (men also produce estogens, but naturally in much smaller amounts than women).

Di-indolylmethane is currently being utilized to treat infections caused by the human papilloma virus, including cervical dysplasia, which is a pre-cancerous lesion.

It is recognized as a suppressor of inflammation and is being studied for use in a variety of viral and bacterial infections.

Glucosinolates are compounds that contain sulfur and nitrogen. If consumed in large amounts, they can cause thyroid enlargement, or goiter. However, in smaller amounts they functions to protect against oxidative damage.

Because cruciferous vegetables are varied, they contain different concentrations and combinations of phytonutrients.

Cruciferous vegetables have a protective effect against certain types of cancers including cancers of the stomach, colon, esophagus, lung and breast. Cruciferous vegetables have also been found to be beneficial in prevention of cataracts and macular degeneration, and may also help reduce blood pressure.

Cauliflower

Cauliflower contains high concentrations of vitamin C, K, manganese, and anti-oxidants like beta-carotene, caffeic acid, ferulic acid, quercetin, rutin, kamferol, and beta-cryptoxanthin. It is also a source of omega 3 fatty acid in the form of alpha-linolenic acid (ALA). These components make cabbage a food with significant anti-inflammatory properties. Its content of soluble fiber also produces a beneficial effect on the digestive tract. Degradation of cauliflower produces compounds called sulforaphane, and glucoraphanin, which are other phytonutrients. Sulforaphane works in preventing overgrowth of the bacterium Helicobacter pylori, which are the bacteria responsible for causing gastric reflux and gastric ulcers.

Cabbage

There are different varieties of cabbage including red, green and Savoy. All of these contain specific phytonutrients called glucosinolates, one of which is sinigrin. Sinigrin is a chemical component that has been shown in research studies to be beneficial in the prevention of cancers of the bladder, colon and prostate. Another compound also found in cabbage is indole-3-carbinol, which has DNA repairing properties and has been used in the prevention of cancer cell development. To get the most of these natural phytonutrients, it is recommended that all varieties of cabbage be consumed, as again, each variety will contain different phytonutrients, in different combinations and concentrations.

Fresh cabbage juice has been used as a tonic to help the healing of gastric ulcers and in some European countries for decades. A paste made from cabbage has been used as an ointment that when applied to inflamed areas of the body, produces an anti-inflammatory effect. Like other cruciferous vegetables, when consumed in large quantities, it can produce a goiter and cause hypothyroidism.

Cabbage is a great source of vitamin K and C, fiber and the amino acid glutamine (an amino acid characterizes by anti-inflammatory properties).

Broccoli

Broccoli also contains a very high concentration of sulforaphane, a natural phytonutrient that stimulates the body's production of carcinogen destroying enzymes.

In addition, it contains phytonutrients, such as gluconasturtian, glucobrassicin and glucoraphanin, which are compounds useful in removing bodily waste and helps in the process of detoxification.

It also contains kaempferol, which is a potent anti-inflammatory flavanoid. Isothiocyanate compounds are responsible for down regulating and shutting off components of the inflammatory system.

Broccoli is a great source of vitamin C, A, K, as well as folate and fiber. It also is a non-animal source of omega 3's.

Kale

Kale is another vegetable with a high concentration of vitamin A, K, C, as well as lutein, and calcium. Like the other cruciferous vegetables mentioned, kale also contain sulforaphane and indole-3-carbinol, which help prevent the development of some cancer cells.

Kale is a source of anti-inflammatory and anti-cancer phytonutrients in the form of glucosinolates, carotenoids and flavonoids.

Carotenoids consist of lutein and beta-carotene, while flavonoids, consist of kaemferol, quercetin and 45 different types of other phytonutrients, all of which have an anti-oxidant effect at the cellular level. Kale has been shown to reduce the cancer risks for cancers of the bladder, prostate, breast, ovary and colon and is currently undergoing studies to look for clinical application.

Collard Greens

Contain high concentration of vitamins C, K, A, as well as manganese, folate and soluble fiber. Collard greens also contain 3,3 'di-indolilmetano,—potent immune modulator with anti-viral, anti-cancer and anti-bacterial effects. Antioxidants found in the leaves of the cabbage, include caffeic acid, ferulic acid, quercetin, and kaemferol, which are also a good source of omega 3 fatty acids.

Radish

The radish has existed for at least 3,000 years. It comes in different varieties, colors and sizes, depending on its class and method used in it is cultivation. Radishes are rich in ascorbic acid, folic acid, vitamin B6, riboflavin, magnesium, copper, calcium and potassium.

It contain sulfa-like compounds, which are beneficial for the digestive tract and the functions of the liver and gallbladder, as well as in the production of bile.

Horseradish

Is a root plant that comes from the family of wasabi and mustard.

Like other cruciferous vegetables, horseradish contains many phytonutrients including sinigrin, a crystalline glucoside form of allyl isothiocyanate.

It is sinigrin, which gives horseradish its strong odor. This food also contains potassium, calcium, vitamin C, magnesium and phosphorus. Mustard oil, which contains anti-bacterial properties, is found in horseradish as well. In medicine it is used as a stimulant, laxative, diuretic and antiseptic.

Brussels Sprouts

Among the cruciferous vegetables, brussel sprouts have the highest concentration of sulforaphanes—a natural component of the plant that has been shown to have potent anti-cancer properties. Is also high in vitamin A and C, as well as a compound called indole-3-carbinol (recognized as a substance that helps with DNA repair and that blocks the development of cancer cells).

Consumption of brussel sprouts has been shown to inhibit the growth of Helicobacter pylori—the bacteria that causes duodenal and gastric ulcers (Galan MV, Kishan AA, Silverman AL (August 2004). Dig Dis Sci. 49 (7-8): 1088-90.

When applied topically, sulforaphane has also been shown to limit the damage caused by UV radiation. Brussels sprouts are also a rich source of protein.

Water

No anti-inflammatory type diet would be complete without mentioning water.

This is because over 60 to 70% of the human body weight is composed of water. There is no substance as essential for normal metabolic processes as clean drinking water.

We are fortunate that in the United States, most of our water is potable (clean and safe to drink).

In many parts of the world, the quality and quantity of available drinking water is scarce or nonexistent.

This, in the 21st century!!!

It may be hard to believe, but the ancient Romans had a better quality of drinking water that half of the world's population today. (www.water.org).

The recommended daily amount of water to drink can be confusing. There are even on-line water requirement calculators one can utilize to help calculate a more accurate water replacement amount.

Some recommend 6 to 8 glasses a day, but of what size container? The medical literature lists eight, 8-ounce glasses of water a day, but I have heart patients with weak heart muscles (cardiomyopathy), that could develop congestive heart failure and end up in the hospital by drinking this amount. All the quoted numbers are a generalization, as water consumption will vary depending on various factors. These include; the persons body weight, age, ambient temperature, activity level and other physiologic considerations, as all of these factors can cause us to loose water through sweat and evaporation.

In general, a person requires 1 to 7 liters of water a day depending on their size, level of physical activity and environmental temperature. Another way to calculate your daily water requirements is to take your weight (in pounds) and divide it by half. The resulting figure is your daily water intake recommendation in ounces. For example, someone who weighs 120 pounds requires about 60 ounces of water a day.

Water is part of an anti-inflammatory diet because it is essential to the process of eliminating waste and toxic substances produced by the body on a daily basis.

Water also helps people lose weight by helping suppress hunger and by aiding in burning calories.

Several studies have recently shown that water is needed and used to burn calories. People who drink at least 8 glasses of water a day burned more calories than those that drank less quantity.

According to a recent study conducted by Virginia Tech University, after a 12 week trial, overweight and obese volunteers who drank 16 ounces of water before each meal, lost on average of 15.5 pounds, compared to 11 pounds of weight loss for those who did not drink water before each meal (44% more weight loss simply by drinking water before each meal!). This weight loss was explained based on the fact that the water drinkers consumed in average of 75 fewer calories with each meal (Brenda M. Davy Journal of the American Dietetic Association, Vol. 108, issue 7, pages 1236-1239. July 2008).

It is interesting to recognize that sometimes the hunger we feel may be the body simply asking for water.

A large percentage of people regularly confuse being thirsty with being hungry. This happens because <u>the hormones in the digestive system that stimulates the brains hunger center are similar to hormones that alert us to thirst.</u> Because it is difficult to sometimes distinguish between these stimuli, <u>we often seek out food and eat, when in fact it, we are thirsty and all we need is to drink water.</u> The next time you are feeling hungry, before reaching for a donut, drink some cold water instead, as it will be filling and may satisfy your cravings.

I want to take a moment to share with you something that I found really interesting. In traditional Chinese medicine, the drinking of cold or ice water while eating a warm meal or hot food is considered to be undesirable because it goes against the entire philosophy of balance, or Yin and Yang.

A hot or warm meal functions to warm up the body and soul, creating a particular state. Drinking a cold beverage provides a completely opposite temperature that has the effect of shocking the digestive system potentially throwing it out of balance. This can then lead to digestive distress and disease.

This is why traditionally a warm or hot beverage, such as saki or tea has been the typical drink of choice when eating traditional Chinese meals.

One of my distinguished professors of Chinese medicine and acupuncture I was taught by, Dr. Fu, Di, pointed out that one reason why Westerners are overweight has to do with the fact that we drink cold water and other cold beverages with our meals. It is this temperature difference and imbalance that allows cold to hinder the smooth flow of the spleen energy, (should be very active while we eat), needed for transforming and transporting nutrients. This slowing down of the digestive function, can in turn contribute to weight gain.

Remember that in Chinese and Ayurdevic medical practice, the body, mind and soul are all interconnected and work in unison.

Yin and Yang, which is a concept of polarity teaches one that to maintain health, all the body's processes have to be working in harmony and be in a state of balance.

When you eat a hot meal, the core of the body is able to receive, extract and properly use the nutrients. The metabolic processes are functioning in a proper, ideal state. By drinking and ingesting a drink that is opposite in temperature, the harmonious digestive process is thrown out of balance. This causes a disturbance, a shock, and a trauma to the body, resulting in an imbalance that can result in many digestive disorders. The simultaneous application of two opposite polarities as reflected in opposing temperature resulting in disease.

Even though the study of traditional Chinese medicine is a lifelong endeavor and I am a beginner, I find that there is much validity in the health concepts of this ancient yet relevant medical thought and practice.

My personal story

On occasion, when I consult patients on smoking cessation and the importance of physical activity and dietary change, they graciously allow me to finish speaking but then look at me tell me that I don't understand how difficult it is for them to change their behavior. They apparently are under the false assumption that anyone with a medical degree must be free of similar bad habits.

Let me tell you that physicians are like anyone else. Some may have a chip on their shoulder, and have huge egos, or are jerks who believe that the world revolves around them, but the great majority of us are very much like you. We are simple, down to earth people concerned about our family, health and wellbeing, just like everyone else.

When it comes to some of my personal bad habits, many would be surprised to learn that for many years I used to rarely drink water.

Until about a few years ago, I drank a liter of diet soda every day. I never drank water—only diet soda. Diet Pepsi or Diet

Coke, it did not matter either, I got which ever was cheaper or on sale.

If you were to come over to my home, you could find about 20, liter size bottles of diet cola in the garage, bought on sale.

Day after day, year after year, I continued to drink diet soda, even while I knew that this behavior on a long-term basis could not possibly be healthy. I was addicted and in denial.

Like many, I rationalized that since diet soft drink is 98 % water, I was basically drinking water. In addition, since it was diet soda, without calories, I had convinced myself I was actually drinking flavored water. It couldn't be so bad, so I just kept drinking it. I had addressed my own concerns with my own delusional belief system.

I chose to ignore the fact that that soft drinks and all soda is carbonated water, crated by the addition of chemicals like carbon dioxide that cause the carbonation and is replete with artificial everything, from sugars in the form of high fructose corn syrup, to flavors and preservatives. I also ignored the fact that soft drinks also contain caffeine and phosphoric acids that are known to bind with calcium and magnesium. Some believe that it is this component that may be associated with, and cause reduced bone density as well as an increase in bone fracture risk (although there is conflicting results).

If you've ever poured a soda on the contacts of a car battery, you can see how this interaction makes the soda start to foam on contact and the corrosion and the chemical buildup on the terminals dissolve away. This occurs as a result of the chemical reactions that occur between the two. And despite this visual and the little voice inside my head and my wife's louder voice telling me otherwise, I still continued to drink diet soda instead of water.

This just goes to show you we can all at like idiots at any given time. Even doctors with credentials, lots of education and analytical minds, are still capable of forming illogical conclusions based on erroneous and perhaps delusional beliefs. Illogical thinking, I believe many people can to relate to.

How the story ends is that during one of the lectures at the University of Arizona, Center for Integrative Medicine where I was completing a Fellowship, behavioral nutritionist, Joy Gurgevich, showed slides comparing the behavior of red blood cells in individuals who drank water and those who drank soda. The slide showing the blood cells of the soda drinkers demonstrated an increase stickiness or adhesion of the red blood cells to each other, causing a slower transit time, and slower red blood cell movement. This is an abnormal cell movement pattern that is scientifically known as Rouleau effect.

Finally, for the first time, I could understand and see with my own eyes, the potentially harmful effects associated with drinking so much soda. Side effects that I had chosen to ignore.

I found myself re-thinking how something as simple, delicious and innocuous as soda, could make such a physiologic impact on the blood and circulation.

I was ready for a change.

It was a decision that I followed up with action, which is what changing a bad habit is all about.

The first thing I did upon returning from the residential week was to stop drinking diet soda.

A small, simple action, but a very important one that led me down a healthier path.

I think it was Gandhi who said that "our future depends with what we do in the present", and what we do in the present starts with one action that will lead to a road of unlimited possibilities.

So then whenever I felt the desire to drink a diet soda (which was basically throughout the entire day and with each meal), I quickly drank a glass of water to quench the desire for soda.

In a rather short time, I was able to stop the obsession and abuse. In my case, it was not as difficult to do, as I had expected. This is important for anyone who wishes to change an unhealthy habit to recognize. I think we frequently sabotage ourselves even before we attempt to change a behavior. Instead of focusing on the end result and the long-term benefits, we focus on how hard or painful the change may be. This is often the reason for failing at something worthwhile.

Today, years later I am happy to report that I am drinking water and tea. On occasions, I will drink some diet cola, which I still enjoy, but gone are the days of drinking only diet soda.

Another bad habit.

When I started doing my internal medicine residency as a first year intern, we would stay up all night admitting patients and working them up, in order to be able to present the case in morning rounds to our residents and senior medical staff members. This was back at a time when people where being diagnosed with a new, mysterious, lethal disease called AIDS.

I was working in a New York area hospital, and was exposed to all sorts of medical illness and diseases, which I could barely pronounce the year before. Now I was responsible for diagnosing and starting the appropriate treatments on an average of 5 new admissions each night while on call. There were no house staff or resident rules limiting the amount of hours of work allowed at that time, so we worked all night long. If we got lucky, we got an hour or two of uninterrupted rest.

Naturally, anything legal that could keep us up was tried and sought after. One night, after the caffeine rush had subsided, one of the senior members of my house call team, a medical doctor from Norway, who also had a Masters degree in public health, gave me one of his Pall Mall cigarettes. Now I had never smoked before, or heard of this brand. All I remember is that it was one strong cigarette! After taking 2 or 3 puffs, I became lightheaded and felt as though my lungs were being ripped out. My throat was blistered and my coughing so profound that tears where coming out of my eye socket.

But something magical happened. After my respiratory distress had subsided and the double vision had cleared, I got the biggest rush I had ever felt. The buzz was so profound that I was able to stay awake for hours. It was apparently the nicotine stimulant that had produced the effect. I soon found myself "borrowing" cigarettes from my colleagues on a regular basis. We would usually smoke in our small staff lounge located in the hospital, on the same floor as the patient rooms. On occasion, the program director would catches us smoking at the nurses station and ask us to extinguish the cigarette which we would, right on the hospital floor. (This behavior would never be acceptable today, and would most likely lead to intervention or immediate termination).

But, soon enough, I had become addicted and was smoking regularly. I smoked for 10 years and never really had the desire to stop. I was fit, exercised, had no family history of heart disease and my lipid levels were great. Again, I was forming illogical conclusions based on erroneous and perhaps delusional beliefs, but they justified my behavior and so I kept smoking. Besides, I wasn't hurting anyone!

Years later I met my future wife. She was (and still is) beautiful and athletic—a former downhill skier on the Junior Olympics and who enjoyed working out and took spinning classes on a regular basis-(still does). I wanted to be able to impress her someday by joining her in a spinning class, so I decided to take a class and see what it was all about. I figured that since I was working out with weights and considered myself to be in good shape, that it would be sort of fun.

I took a class.

Let me tell you, I soon thought I was gonna die. And this was only after the first 10 minutes of the spinning class, during the warm up phase!

My legs slowly began to feel like they were burning, because I was out of shape. I tried to get my legs to go one way, they chose to go the other way. I was tired, winded and short of breath. I pretended to enjoy the pace, but was actually grimacing in discomfort. I soon left, by pretending my beeper had gone off.

That experience was a reality check, and my wake up call. It was also the start of my desire to quit smoking.

Again, I knew better, but I have learned that some people will make the correct lifestyle choices only when they are ready for it. Hopefully, the changes will occur before any permanent harm comes to their health.

After about 10 years of addiction and 3 attempts at quitting, I was able to stop smoking many years ago. So, when patients tell me I just don't understand how hard it is to change an unhealthy habit, the reality is that I do. Likewise, many other healthcare providers also understand you and your situation, as many of have had similar experiences.

I have had to learn how to balance high fat foods that I enjoy and that most of us grew up with (fast foods and comfort foods), by balancing these foods with healthier food choices.

When I realized I had gained weight, I took a action to correct it.

I was not motivated enough to re-join a gym. Did not want the hassle of driving through traffic, finding a parking space, an empty locker and available equipment to use. I knew I would find excuses to not go. Instead, I bought myself a treadmill that was on sale. I make time to use it 20 minutes, 5 days a week while watching the news or Golden Girls re-runs. I also bought a pedometer and try to walk 10,000 steps a day, to try to stay healthy.

I lost 20 lbs and re-toned my body, simply by walking on the treadmill. I changed my focus, removed any roadblock or obstacle I would have otherwise placed myself, and just changed a habit.

My most important reality check is however seeing the poor condition of hospitalized patients, as well as treating office patients on a daily basis who are suffering from various stages of easily controllable diseases. The increase numbers of younger aged patients opened my eyes to just how fortunate I am to be in good health.

In addition to healthier food choices and regular exercise, I have also been taking an omega 3 capsule, a multi-vitamin and a 81-milligram aspirin (baby dose), in the morning before I go to work.

I only mention my story to share with you the fact that no matter how impressive someone appears to be or how many credentials they may have or position of power they hold, we all go through the same struggles.

Gradually, with one change at a time, you too can achieve more than you can imagine. It just takes one step in the positive direction.

Final Thoughts

I hope you have found this book interesting and that you may have learned something new. Indeed, my reason for writing it was so that I could share with my patients what I had just learned during my Integrative Medicine Fellowship. Most importantly, the role our everyday nutrition and diet plays as potential cause of disease, as well as a its relevance in preserving our health.

As doctors we are always advising our patients to avoid sodium, limit fat ingestion and reduce calories. Recommendations that constitute pretty much the standard suggestions when it comes to our knowledge on nutrition. You can ask 5 different doctors for dietary advice and there's a good chance you'll get 5 different responses, all pretty much revolving around the same recommendation. And this is because a curriculum in nutrition is not taught in medical school or in residencies and knowledge is limited.

Food is medicine. Like any medicine it can help us when used appropriately but it can also cause harm when abused or used inappropriately.

The impact that nutrition plays on our health and wellness as well as the fact that it is the one thing we can control without much effort, makes our daily diet and the type and quality of foods we eat one of the most important modifiable factors we have at our control.

Sadly, we have become a medical system and a society addicted to drugs. And why not, when we continuously get bombarded by 30 second commercials that reinforce our need for drugs to find happiness, wellbeing and relief from everything that ails us.

Truth is we have been killing ourselves by way of our mouth, specifically by our poor food choices.

We eat too much of the wrong foods that are of poor quality. We do so because it is abundant, and affordable. Increasingly we use food not so much for nourishment, but rather as a go to when our emotions dictate it.

Food has become our escape, our past time, our friend, our lover and confidant. Many people eat without even being hungry. Our lives seem to revolve around food.

As a result, portion sizes have increased by 100% since the 1970's. The consumption of meats, sweeteners and calories have all, likewise increased, while at the same time physical activity has decreased. Most importantly we shifted from being a country that ate healthier foods intermittently, to one that is continuously eating foods containing saturated fats, sugars and processed foods loaded with chemicals and other substances that were never meant to be in food in the first place.

We have a Congress and politicians at the National and State level that contribute to this country's epidemics of obesity, diabetes, and other chronic illnesses, by the incredibly thoughtless and even outright stupid decisions they make. It seems that many of them are more interested in keeping the status quo and in pleasing their corporate donors, than in looking after the wellbeing of the people they are supposed to serve.

Pizza, considered a vegetable.

Subsidies and tax breaks for industrial food conglomerates.

Eliminating physical education class in many school systems.

No incentives or programs to help grow fresh, organic fruits, vegetables and products.

No help in making healthy food choices more affordable.

Politicians at the State level who question the effectiveness and need for health prevention programs, suggesting that now is not the time to spend money on prevention of disease.

With these few examples, how can politicians claim to be working on resolving our healthcare crisis? Passing legislation allowing pizza to be considered a vegetable is not only embarrassing it is insulting to all Americans. It defies logic especially when people are developing more chronic illnesses that lead to increased healthcare costs, as a result of our lifestyle.

These few examples help to illustrate how Congress and some of our elected officials play politics and why they share a large part of the blame for our country's health crisis. Our nations deteriorating health and continued increase in healthcare expenditures should be treated as a threat to our National security and addressed as such.

Likewise, those of us in healthcare need to do a better job in educating and informing people about the important role food has on our health.

A role that is in our hands to control, and in so doing, help delay or prevent the onset of many illnesses caused by poor dietary choices.

We are better able to understand the significant relationship that exists between the foods we eat on a regular basis and our states of health.

After being absorbed, food alters the normal bodily functions. Converting food into energy causes an increase in cellular, oxidative stress.

If we eat reduced portions, intermittently and occasionally, this stress is beneficial. When we eat excessively and continuously, in the manner that our society has been doing for decades, it can damage a cell's DNA, both directly and indirectly.

As we have been eating more quantities of nutrient poor food, we have gotten fatter. Fat tissue in turn, produces several hormones as well as other pro-inflammatory substances.

All of the added fats, preservatives and chemicals added to many foods during their manufacture and processing, also contribute in developing pro-inflammatory states.

As a result, chronic inflammation gradually develops. This chronic inflammation caused by poor quality foods and unhealthy nutrition, has become a common underlying factor in the development of chronic illness.

Chronic illnesses, that although diverse share in common underlying chronic inflammation.

We went from an active society, accustomed to eating larger amounts of fresh fruits and vegetables, with occasional red meat, (similar to our ancestral biology), to a society on the go, consuming convenience foods that are highly processed and loaded with calories, sugars and fats.

The good news is that although it has been slow in coming, more Americans are recognizing the importance of nutrition and food in maintaining health.

Many are seeking healthier food choices and trying to maintain healthier lifestyles.

The increasing cost associated with healthcare has been an important factor for the changing trends.

Popular culture also plays an important role, by opening the eyes of many Americans, to the sad reality of how unhealthy and overweight our nation has become.

One of the most popular prime-time television shows puts extremely obese people though grueling workouts and teaches them (as well as the viewer) about healthy eating habits.

There has been a steady rise in the number of similar television shows, as well as cooking shows that emphasize healthier, lower calorie meals, that have also helped increased awareness.

Corporations have taken note and are making much needed changes in areas of nutrition.

Fast-food establishments are offering healthier variety of food selections. Some offer oatmeal, salads, grilled chicken breast sandwiches, and one of the largest fast-food franchises, the option of vegetables to accompany their children's meals.

To keep up with the demands of the public, a national chicken manufacturer recently began advertising their line of healthier chicken products, claiming their chickens are raised, free-range style.

Even natural sugar is making a comeback, as it is making a return, replacing high fructose corn syrup in many food items. These are healthy small steps pointed in the right direction.

We have been abusing ourselves for decades by eating excessive amounts of nutrient poor foods. Improving our food selection is the easiest change all of us can make to improve our quality of life.

You don't need to have a degree in health, but you do need to use common sense.

We could reduce this Nation's healthcare costs, and the associated costs spent on medications and pharmaceuticals, simply by eating healthier foods and making better food choices.

Changing what we eat CAN change our health.

This is the message we need to get out and as individuals and a society we can't afford to wait or depend on Washington to take the lead and do what is right.

Instead of consuming pre-packaged, processed, foods and snacks packed with chemical preservatives, we need to start eating less processed, more natural foods from all 3 macronutrients food groups. We also need to reduce our portion sizes and increase our physical activity levels.

While pre-packaged, celebrity endorsed weight loss meals work for some, I don't get very excited or impressed by any of them. While we frequently see celebrities that achieve spectacular weight loss and look great, I wonder if there have been others who were not as successful. Celebrities who failed to loose the desired weight and whose commercials and testimonials we therefore never got to see, but who nonetheless got paid hundreds of thousands or millions of dollars for their time.

I am more concerned about the amount of preservatives some of these meals contain, especially the meals that do not need refrigeration. Foods that were manufactured and prepared weeks before, that can be kept in their container until used.

They are of reduced calories and portion sizes, and thus they are easy and convenient. If these work for you, than it is worth a try. I would however recommend that you buy healthier foods and consuming smaller portions.

Any diet that is of lower calorie (a diet we can make ourselves), along with eating smaller portions more frequently throughout the day and that incorporates exercise will result in weight loss.

To illustrate this, just a few days ago, one of the larger of the national, celebrity endorsed weight loss plans started airing their new commercial. It stared a woman who had lost 100 pounds eating their food. In addition, she mentioned that she had also been running 7 miles a day.

It doesn't take an "expert" to figure this one out that anyone who runs 7 miles a day, will loose weight and keep it off. You could eat a large pepperoni pizza each day, while running 7 miles a day, and you too would loose weight. So, was it in fact, a particular diet brand that caused the weight loss, or the lower calorie, smaller portioned meals and exercise that resulted in the weight loss? It's obvious.

We need to stop believing in all the "miracle" weight loss fantasies claimed in the tabloids, magazines, infomercials, and sold on TV.

THERE IS NO MAGIC WEIGHT LOSS FORMULA. (Yet).

Loosing weight requires work. Maintaining a healthy diet is less challenging once we recognize the great variety available to us. Changing how and what you eat should not be a burden. A gradual transition from unhealthy processed foods to more nutritious, unprocessed natural foods and a reduction in the amount of processed food is all that is suggested. Whatever you do, don't obsess over how and what to eat.

There is no magic diet, magic weight loss pills, weight loss potions, or devices that you wear that will make you eat less and loose weight, for life.

Remedies that provide a quick and limited loss of weight is not what we should be seeking.

Be cautious in believing any health benefit claims that are made in order to sell a product.

This is especially true of claims made by so-called experts. It seems that we can find experts in every field. Many of whom are paid to say exactly whatever they get paid to say.

Trust, but verify.

It is up to each one of us to work at maintaining and regaining the good health most of us were born with.

Health is everyone's problem.

Suggestions.

We need to start reading labels to become familiar with what we are consuming. Compare, become informed and verify what is being said about all products sold.

Continuously ask questions. Look up the responses you received. You must become your own advocate and become knowledgeable when it comes to nutrition.

Exercise should be a part of everyone's day.

The older one is, the more important exercise becomes. As previously mentioned, exercise is indicated as part of ALL popular weight loss diets. Exercise does more than just burn calories it also produces many beneficial health effects. Reason why it is important for everyone, regardless of body weight, to try and make it a part of your day.

I consider exercise to be as important a <u>medication,</u> as nutrition. If you have enough time to take a shower, you have enough time to do some exercise.

We need to start becoming more aware of the foods we eat. Doing this should not be a chore or a burden it should be fun and interesting.

Start by reading nutrition labels.

Try to increase the consumption of less processed, whole foods and foods that are as fresh as possible.

Because of their healthier, highly nutritive content and the time and effort that goes into their cultivation, some organic-type produce and naturally raised meat products may be slightly more costly than the mass-produced commercially farmed foods. There are certain things, however, we can do to minimize their costs.

Buy in bulk

Buying in bulk allows you to split and costs with friends or family members. You can find sales on all items including organic, and healthy food products. You can find olive oil, breads, fruits, vegetables, lean meats, beans and other healthy food items on sale. My wife and I usually buy 12-grain bread when they are at a buy 1, get 1 sale, and then freeze a loaf.

Once thawed, the bread is just as fresh as when we bought it, without any change in moisture, texture or consistency. I recommend you try this at home.

Reduced price sales

Take advantage of in-season produce offers. In South Florida, you can find a major grocery store frequently offering 3 containers of strawberries for $5. Other fruits like blueberries, blackberries and other fresh locally grown fruits, are also frequently similarly put on sale. What we don't eat right away, we freeze. They may not all be all organic but at least they are fruits with natural sugars, fibers, nutrients and phytonutrients, essential for a healthy, balanced diet.

Like fruits, vegetables from across the color spectrum can also frequently be found on sale. Again, try buying in bulk if possible, especially when in season and share among friends and family members. Many of these items can be stored in different ways, preferably frozen, for use at a later time.

Buy local !!

By buying produce from local area farms and growers, you get fresher, better quality produce. Local produce is less costly, because there is a shorter time period from cultivation to the table, as well as shorter transportation distance and time.

Obtaining produce from local suppliers also eliminates the need for processing and preservatives.

I was pleasantly surprised to see a national food chain that specialize in organic and whole foods, have a large section dedicated to locally produced produce. One particular store in South Miami, had melons, strawberries, and all a large assortment of fresh vegetables that were grown and produced locally. Even more surprising was the cheaper prices of these locally grown organic products, over the mass-produced variety, shipped in from thousands of miles away.

This goes to show us that we shouldn't make assumptions. Just because a store specializes in organic and natural food products, it doesn't mean all items will automatically be more expensive.

Farmers markets

Farmers markets are another great way to buy locally grown and affordable produce. Most cities and towns have their own version of a farmers market, held periodically at various times throughout the year. The available selection and variety, depending on the area of the country you live in, is often times greater than at some of the larger food stores. In Miami Dade County, the health department and the Consortium for a Healthy Miami-Dade (www.healthymiamidade.org) are taking the initiative and lead in increasing awareness to the importance of nutrition and physical activity. One of the current programs is in helping establish farmers markets in various communities in S. Florida that does not have easy access to healthy, fresh vegetables and fruits.

Gardening anyone??

Plant your own garden! Why not plant your own Victory gardens like they did back in the 40's and 50's?

While I realize that many may not have access to large open spaces to plant gardens, those that do should try it. There is nothing more rewarding (and healthier), than eating something you had a hand in creating that is pesticide and chemical free.

In addition, it is a fun way to get out, get some sun and spend some time with your kids or by yourself and with nature. Even people who live in apartments can buy basil or rosemary plants to give any routine meal, your own special personal touch.

It is encouraging to see reports in the news of school kids being taught about the importance of a healthy diet and then given the time and space needed, to actually start their own gardens on school property.

What is old is becoming new again, and a return to healthier food choices is the first step to a healthier society.

Other suggestions that may help improve your nutrition.

1. Consider taking omega 3 supplements daily. While a diverse, balanced diet contains minerals and vitamins, it will not supply enough of this beneficial fatty acid. The recommended daily dose is 900-1000mg of the EPA/DHA component. If you go over, it doesn't matter. You need however, more than 900mg a day. Omega 3 is not included in typical multi-vitamin supplements. I would also not recommend combination omega supplements that contain any other omegas in the formulation. There is no need to take supplements containing omega 3, 6 and 9 in the same formulations. We eat too much omega 6 (pro-inflammatory) and too little omega 3 (anti-inflammatory).

2. Start small. Don't try to change a lifetime of bad eating habits or unhealthy lifestyle in a couple of days. This will only lead to frustration and disinterest.

Make small changes every day and stick with it. This may eventually lead to a life long transformation. What may seem to you to be a small and insignificant change, will lead to many other healthy changes.

3. Eat slowly. It takes approximately 20 minutes for the brain to think you are full.

4. Eat half of what is on your plate and take the rest home.

5. Drink water when you feel hungry.

6. Use smaller sized plates to help you control portion sizes.

7. Keep the food in the kitchen out of sight. This way you won't be continuously tempted to eat when you are not hungry.

8. Skip the frequent bacon cheeseburger or pizza. Instead pack a turkey or other healthy lunch.

9. Buy a pedometer. This device attaches to your belt or you can put it in a pocket. It counts the number of steps you walk in a day. They can cost from as little as $5 to over $50, so you can see how much you walk (or don't walk) during the day. I use one that cost $10 and it works fine. You'll be amazed at how little most of us walk during our day.

10. Keep reading and educating yourself on nutrition, healthy lifestyle choices and stress and anxiety control. Remember that many physicians and healthcare providers don't fully understand the impact that nutrition has on health.

A patient of mine mentioned that he had been successfully treated for prostate cancer. When I recommended he eat tomatoes, tomato products and cruciferous vegetables because of the anti-cancerous phytochemicals they contain, he told me that his prostate specialist, (a university professor), had told him to avoid tomatoes and other vegetables because they could cause bladder discomfort.

This is an example of the huge disconnect that exist in American medicine. As physicians, we can easily offer different treatment recommendations, especially when it comes to nutrition recommendations. Some of these may even be detrimental and confusing for our patients, who are already receiving so many mixed messages.

11. Don't worry over how much you weigh. Some people get real stressed if they don't loose an x amount of pounds in a certain amount of time. Keep eating healthy foods and doing routine exercise. This is what you should strive for, not how much weight did or did not come off.

Pounds are only a number that you should use as a guide. It is not who you are.

In addition, training with weights tend to create muscle mass. Muscle weighs more than fat. After training with weights you may increase slightly in weight as a positive effect. Muscle also burns more calories than non-muscle tissue.

12. The food pregnant women eat may impact and influence the future eating habits of the baby, so it is crucial that pregnant women eat healthy.

You owe it to yourself to ask your healthcare provider or registered dietician for information on healthy food choices and lifestyle choices. There are so many different areas of medicine that are new and interesting that it makes it easy for me to enjoy continued learning about disease prevention and wellness.

I hope you too can find this joy in learning.

Food for life.

I end as I began . . .

"The doctor of the future will prescribe no medicine, but will want to educate their patients in the care of the body, proper diet, and disease prevention."

~ Thomas A. Edison

About the author

Jorge Bordenave is a 3rd generation physician who grew up in a household where each evening he would hear stories of wellness and miracles. There was no doubt he too would follow in the footsteps of healers.

Concerned over the lack of reliable, up to date healthcare information available to the diverse Hispanic communities across the United States, he is the only current US trained and practicing physician to write directly for Spanish speakers across the United States, Central and South America as well as Spain.

Dr. Bordenave completed his first residency, in Internal Medicine, in New York and Chicago. This was followed by a Clinical, Invasive and Nuclear Cardiology Fellowship at Mt. Sinai Medical Center.

Interested in many fields of medicine and an avid scuba diver, he continued his medical education by taking multiple dive and hyperbaric medicine courses. He is a graduate of the National Oceanographic and Atmospheric Administration physicians dive medicine program. Currently, he is the only NOAA/UHMS certified medical examiner of divers in South Florida.

He is a Screen Actors Guild approved physician who has been the production physician for many of the television series and motion pictures filmed in South Florida, over the last 15 years.

He is currently in private practice in South Florida and a public speaker and educator to community groups on topics of health and prevention, in both English and Spanish.

He found time to enroll at the George Washington University School of Business, where has 6 remaining credits to complete his healthcare MBA.

His most rewarding medical educational experience was in completing a third fellowship in Integrative Medicine at the University of Arizona Center for Integrative Medicine.

"The fellowship reminded me that physicians are still healers and that oftentimes healing is accomplished simply by just listening to the patient and acknowledging them as an individual. A concept that is foreign to the way medicine is practiced today in the United States, where ordering tests and prescribing pills has become the "standard of excellence".

Wanting to learn more in depth about areas of complementary medicine, he regularly seeks out and takes medical courses.

Recently, he completed additional course work in acupuncture and Chinese medicine at the University of Miami.

A lifelong learner and interested in issues of public health, he applied and has been accepted to the

Johns Hopkins Bloomberg School of Public Health.

Dr. Bordenave has been recipient of several awards, including the NCQA recognition awards (2007-2010, 2010-2013) for excellence in medical care of cardiac and diabetic patients.

He has averaged over 200 CME credit hours of continuing medical education per year and is an active participant in the Florida Medicare Quality Improvement Organization (FMQAI).

He is a graduate of the Harvard Quality Colloquium.

He is a voting member of the New York Academy of Science and member of several National medical/scientific organizations. Included are; the American Heart Association—member of the Nutrition, Physical Activity and Metabolism council, the American College of Cardiology, the Underwater Hyperbaric Medical Society, American Dietetic Association and American Association for the Advancement of Science to name a few.

He is a Fellow of the American College of Physicians, Fellow of the American Board of Quality Assurance, and Fellow of the American Healthcare Institute.

A lifelong educator, he is currently an active, voluntary Clinical Associate Professor of Medicine at the Herbert Wertheim Medical College at Florida International University and a lecturer in cardiology for the Family Practice and Internal Medicine residency programs at a South Florida teaching hospital. A physician mentor, he regularly has medical students and residents rotating with him.

He serves on the continuing medical education committee at Palmetto General Hospital in Miami, is the physician member of the Performance Improvement committee at Larkin Community Hospital and member of the peer review and quality improvement committee for a large managed care organization based in South Florida.

He is a physician volunteer for the Liga Contra el Cancer, the San Juan Bosco church free clinic, as well as speaker for cancer support groups in areas of nutrition and mind body healing. He is a member of the Consortium for a Healthier Miami-Dade, working with the Miami Dade Health department and other stakeholders in trying to improve the health of South Floridians.

His interests include, prevention, complimentary medicine, traditional Chinese medicine and studying healthcare systems from around the world.

His passion however remains in patient education specifically in the importance of nutrition and physical activity in disease prevention.

He tries to empower, teach and motivate patients, to be able to take control of their own health.

When not learning, he enjoys traveling, photography, cooking, water sports, writing and staying active.

He will continue to target and direct his health education and other health and medical writings for the Spanish speaking populations, as it is currently the largest underserved segment of society when it comes to health education.

Most importantly, he will continue to remind patients of the body's innate ability to heal itself, without the need of toxic drugs or chemicals.

Other Books by Dr. Bordenave

La dieta anti-inflamatoria

Cambie Su Dieta, Cambie Su Salud

Your Healthcare Manual

Su Manual de la Salud

Understanding Fibromyalgia

In medicine, as it has always been, less is more.

INDEX